THE DYNA-STEP CHALLENGE

GW00536427

ALSO BY HILARY ATKINSON & ANDRE E DEANE
THE DYNA-BAND CHALLENGE

THE DYNA-STEP CHALLENGE

THE NEW STEP WORKOUT FOR HIGH-ENERGY FITNESS

**HILARY ATKINSON
& ANDRÉE DEANE**

Published in 1993 by Vermilion Arrow
an imprint of Ebury Press
Random House UK Ltd
20 Vauxhall Bridge Road
London SW1V 2SA

1 3 5 7 9 10 8 6 4 2

A catalogue record for this book
is available from the British Library

Photography by Jeff Kaine
Designed by Roger Walker

Printed and bound in Great Britain
by Cox & Wyman Ltd, Reading Berkshire

ISBN 0 09 929591 1

WARNING

If you have a medical condition, or are
pregnant, the exercises described in this
book should not be followed without first
consulting your doctor. All guidelines and
warnings should be read carefully, and the
author and publisher can not accept
responsibility for injuries or damage arising
out of a failure to comply with the same.

Contents

INTRODUCTION 7

1 WELCOME TO STEPPING 15

2 WHY STEP? 19

3 ABOUT THE CHALLENGE 27

4 STEP SAFELY 33

5 WARMING UP 45

6 NEW STEPPER'S CHALLENGE 74

7 ADVANCED DYNA-STEP CHALLENGE 125

8 TIGHT TUMS AND HEALTHY BACKS 180

9 COOLING DOWN 196

10 SPECIAL STEPPERS 206
Pregnant Women, Children, Mature Steppers

APPENDIX: Step Summary 216

Special Dyna-Step and Video Offer 224

This book is dedicated to the thousands of readers who took up the Dyna-Band Challenge and whose many letters of support and encouragement have inspired me to write this new Dyna-Step Challenge.

Introduction

From being an ordinary mother and wife with an interest in exercise and an overwhelming desire to have a firm, fit body, I have quite suddenly found myself in the exercise business! It's a business that grew out of my despair with the exercise programmes available, and my increasing belief that diets just do not work. Let me stress, until a few years ago, I was a fulltime wife and mother with no fitness experience or expertise. I wanted what most busy women (and men) of today want – a quick, easy and enjoyable form of exercise that produced spectacular benefits – and it was that basic request that spawned Dyna-Bands and its successor, Dyna-Step.

Those of you who are already familiar with the Dyna-Band story will know how these extraordinary pieces of latex revolutionized my life. After witnessing their effects and then experimenting with them in my own exercise programme, I went on to become the sole distributor of Dyna-Bands in the UK and Channel Islands, selling them from my own home. My enthusiasm for Dyna-Bands grew daily. My own noticeably improving figure was testimony to the fact that they really worked, and I found converts in anyone else who tried them. This was fun, easy and effective exercise. How could it fail? Soon enough the press caught on, and the interest generated an enormous response from stockists – a response which has never waned.

At the beginning of 1990, I was approached by Ebury Press, who wanted to publish an exercise book using Dyna-Bands. I needed to find a writer and a fitness consultant to work with – and I found both in the form of Andrée Deane.

Andrée had been using Dyna-Bands in her fitness training classes on a regular basis. Furthermore, I discovered from several people in the fitness profession that she was a highly qualified, respected and well-known lecturer and exercise teacher who was running one of the most successful exercise-teacher training courses in the country. Also important to me was the fact that Andrée was a young mother, so she was aware of the time constraints involved in raising a family and running a household. She would have had a post-natal body to get back into shape, so she would also understand the needs of the many women who had so far found it impossible to regain their former physiques.

Andrée devised a programme of exercises that could be done at home, took minimum time and fuss, and yet still gave quick results. The Dyna-Band programme could be done in ten minutes each day, or twenty, three times a week. The Dyna-Step Challenge offers that same flexibility and simplicity.

The book was an outstanding success, confirming my belief in Dyna-Bands and Andrée herself.

Over the three years since those early days of promoting Dyna-Bands, I have received thousands of letters from exercisers across the nation. It really works! they cried. See the difference! One by one exercisers have discovered what I already knew – that exercise could have miraculous effects, and that it could be done in the comfort of your own home. Dyna-Bands sparked a flurry of interest in exercising among women and men who had more or less given up hope of ever being fit. With those principles in mind, Andrée and I are back with a new and exciting exercise challenge – stepping routines that can be done in very little space, in the minimum of time, and with any level of experience. The challenges in this book are set for anyone – and can be used on any step.

FROM STRETCHING TO STEPPING

It was about two years after I started distributing Dyna-Bands that I noticed a new trend emerging. In America people were stepping on and off little boxes as a form of exercise. They raved about the effects and I began to take an interest.

For exercise to be popular, it has to be easy and show consistent benefits. Stepping offers so much more than most forms of aerobic exercise. Using any kind of music, stepping can be done on your own or in a group. And the biggest advantage is the different ways of doing it. Routines are ever-changing so it's never boring. The up-and-down movement improves co-ordination and grace, and most importantly burns off calories and speeds up the metabolism. It's a fantastic, all-round form of exercise. Even better, stepping can be done anywhere, and on any kind of safe step. I was fascinated by stepping, and the possibilities offered by it.

About the same time my UK stockists started asking if I could supply them with a step – something a little cheaper, and perhaps safer than those already on the market. Stepping was becoming all the rage, and they needed to supply a good step to keep up with the demand. With most of my energy still sunk into Dyna-Bands, I had little time to investigate this new form of exercising. My interest was renewed, however, when I came across the prototype for the Dyna-Step.

It was everything we were looking for. Designed by the leaders of the aerobics field in America, it was built according to the specifications of fitness experts, ironing out all the shortcomings of steps already on the market. Here's what Dyna-Step has to offer:

• A lightweight, easy-to-transport step. Many instructors supply steps for their classes, and lugging around unwieldy and heavy steps is not only time-consuming and inconvenient, but also completely impractical. The Dyna-Step is extremely light – so light that it has encouraged many participants to bring their own steps to class. Even more importantly, the Dyna-Step stacks away neatly in the corner of any room in your house – or it's lightweight enough to lift on top of a cupboard or wardrobe for storage. With a large and bulky step you are much less likely to treat yourself to a spontaneous workout if it's an effort to go outside and get it from the garage or storeroom.

• A less-expensive step. Although the benefits of step exercising speak for themselves, the cost of purchasing the steps for home or class use was prohibitive to many would-be exercisers. Exercise should be affordable, and available to everyone. Dyna-Step ensures that it is, at less than two-thirds the price of most other steps.

• A safe form of exercise. In the first chapter Andrée discusses the dangers of some of the earlier steps on the market. It was essential that we find a step that was stable, user-friendly, designed to prevent injury, and capable of being fixed firmly to the floor to avoid dangerous skidding. Well, the makers of Dyna-Step had thought of everything. Not only is it softer, and therefore more cushioned, than many of the other steps on the market, but it has non-slip pads on the base, to prevent any nasty accidents. Made of the same material as surf boards and archery target boards, Dyna-Step is durable, with enough give to prevent the jarring action that impact exercise can cause. Furthermore, the protective mat or covering attached to the top of the Dyna-Step absorbs a great deal of the impact as you step on to it. Many physiotherapists have approved its shock-absorbent material.

• The step must be height adjustable. Exercisers come in all different shapes and sizes and levels of experience. The step must be safe and accessible for all levels. And Dyna- Step is just that. The Dyna-Step is made up of two blocks – one of five inches and the other of three inches in height. They slot together almost like Lego bricks to make a total height of eight inches. This arrangement can give you a great deal of flexibility when stepping. You can choose to work on a five- or eight-inch step, which caters for all levels of ability. When the two blocks are separated and placed in a T-shape, as illustrated in Chapter 8, it provides a comfortable base on which to lie or sit and perform your conditioning exercises. The Dyna-Step could not be more versatile.

It looked like Dyna-Step was what we were looking for. But there were, of course, some sceptics. How could something so light and insubstantial looking bear up to constant thumping? And was it safe? It was important to me to get it right. The success of Dyna-Bands had given me a reputation of which I could be proud. I had to be absolutely certain that the Dyna-Step was of the same quality and as effective as Dyna-Bands. Again, proof was in the offing. At the health show in London last year, the step was made available for testing and the response was enthusiastic. The Dyna-Step was purchased unreservedly by fitness experts, would-be exercisers and physiotherapists alike. The calls and letters that have flooded in since that time have only served to confirm our belief in Dyna-Step. The overwhelming consensus is this: Dyna-Step is problem free.

A STEP IN THE RIGHT DIRECTION

The cardiovascular effects of stepping, which Andrée describes in the first chapters, are outstanding. And unlike most forms of cardiovascular workout, stepping is not repetitive and dull. People do feel the quite amazing benefits – and see them, too. Women especially rave about the effects on their lower body and tummy. Even if you are very overweight, stepping can be a safe and comfortable form of aerobic exercise, without the dangers that high-impact exercise can offer.

I had always had a well-rounded exercise programme with Dyna-Bands, and I was enthralled by my new, firm body. Cardiovascular exercise was covered by my energetic walking sessions – primarily to collect and deliver my daughter to school. Unfortunately, she soon reached an age where it was unseemly for mum to be seen anywhere near her or in the vicinity of the school and I began to miss the exercise offered by those walks. I found myself becoming breathless more easily. Stepping seemed to be the answer. It was quick, effective cardiovascular exercise that I could fit easily into my increasingly busy schedule, and more than that, I discovered that I loved it! What a sense of achievement to master progressively complex and challenging routines. I felt my co-ordination and overall fitness level improve daily.

Many of the letters that I have received about Dyna-Step and Dyna-Bands are from women who have discovered that exercise has changed their lives. Busy housewives, mothers with young families, and working women have little time for exercise classes. Add up the time it takes to pack a bag, drive to the class, get through the class and home again, and it's nearly two or three hours gone from a busy day. Babysitters, or rides have to be arranged. All in all, a lot of effort for a little exercise. The great thing about stepping is that it can be done at home – in even the tiniest living area. There aren't many forms of aerobic exercise that can offer that. And because the step can be easily tucked away and retrieved, you can stop for twenty minutes, do a quick routine, and pop it away again in time for supper. In my daughter's house, her young children use the step to sit on as they watch television!

The increasing popularity of stepping has led to this book being published. It's important to remember that you can use any step for the exercises, as long as it's safe and comfortable. In Chapter 2, Andrée talks more about the kind of step to look for, if you want to hire one, or buy your own. All of the exercises in this book are suitable for any kind of step, so if you've got a step, or can hire one, or borrow from a friend, you are ready to go. You can even try out the routines on the floor.

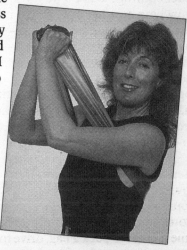

Stepping is the answer to the fitness needs of many many women and men, and without further ado I shall turn you over to Andrée, fitness expert extraordinaire, who is set to challenge you back to peak health and fitness. Good luck! If you enjoy it even half as much as I do, you'll be hooked for life.

HILARY ATKINSON

CHAPTER 1
Welcome to Stepping

I am proud to have been involved in exercise and fitness, both as a participant and an instructor, for the past twelve years; in fact, I have loved every minute of it. I have also spent several years teaching physical education to children in schools so, as you can imagine, I enjoy any form of sport or physical fitness. I also believe that all physical activity, with appropriate modifications, should be available to just about all ages and ability levels.

Most of the exercise classes I teach are now 'step aerobic' classes, which will give you some indication of the popularity of stepping, and I also train other fitness enthusiasts to become instructors. Over the years I have seen fitness products come and go and new types of exercise programmes devised – but a great deal of these new ideas come briefly into vogue only to disappear a short time later. Fitness enthusiasts are always looking for something new mainly because:

- they want their bodies to look fitter and leaner;
- they would like quicker results; and
- their programme needs to be more challenging and fun.

Now that step aerobics has arrived – has it satisfied all of these needs? After following this programme I think that you will agree with me when I say that step aerobics is definitely here to stay. It satisfies all of these needs and more.

I participated in my first step class three years ago in America. There were two hundred of us stomping up and down in an enormous ballroom and, within five minutes, I was hooked – despite the fact that I could barely see the instructor! I could not believe how many different ways there were to get on and off a step! And yet, it was not complicated, everybody seemed to be following quite easily. OK, so every now and then one of us would be up when we were supposed to be down and down when we were supposed to be up – but it didn't matter. You don't bump into each other or make yourself look a total fool like you can do in some dance aerobic classes. Everyone else is concentrating so hard on their own step to the exclusion of everything around them. I felt great during and after the workout. My whole body had been involved effectively in the exercises and I had a great sense of achievement from rising to the challenge. What's more – it was great fun.

In those early stepping days some manufacturers jumped on the step bandwagon, determined to make some quick money. It was for this reason that some of the step boxes on sale left a lot to be desired in terms of safety and durability. Wooden boxes were a firm favourite as they were inexpensive to produce, but they often had sharp edges which could lead to vicious cuts and bruises. Other plastic steps were insubstantial and not geared to consistent jumping on and off. Some steps were barely big enough to hold more than a tiny foot, and many were only available in one height, which would have been too high for the beginner stepper or anyone less than six foot tall! Fortunately, with three years stepping now behind us, instructors have made stricter demands upon the safety and durability of steps. We now have products that are much more suited to the activity, including, of course, the Dyna-Step. In Chapter 2 I discuss the comparative merits of the steps that are available and suggest what you should look for.

Many of the instructors that I have trained have taken to stepping like ducks to water and, not content with just teaching step classes, they participate in as much stepping at home as they possibly can. They become hooked because they can actually see the changes taking place in their body shape, they can feel the improvements to their fitness levels, and they experience the euphoria that a successful exercise programme can provide. These instructors have noticed that their legs, particularly thighs and buttocks, have tightened almost immediately. Their body fat begins to decrease (the flabby abdomen starts to disappear) and they look and feel great! But that's not all – step exercise seems almost addictive. You will find that you will want to conquer more and more step patterns and accept new challenges.

You will want to aim for the Advanced Dyna-Step Challenge (see Chapter 7) to increase your fitness levels and achieve even better results. After your first attempt at the step I am convinced that you will want to try more. Results are so fantastic that all steppers seem to be highly motivated, which means that adherence to the step programme is very good.

How many times have you started a new exercise or diet programme only to become bored or frustrated with it? I am sure that each and every one of us has at some stage in our life given up on a resolution to change our lifestyle in some way. This step programme will challenge and excite you, as well as give you quick results – therefore you are much more likely to stick to it.

So what are you waiting for? Read on through all of the first few chapters of the book, for it is important that you go through the step-safety and warming-up chapters before embarking on either of the step challenges. I know how tempting it is to go straight to the exercises but this would be unwise, particularly if you have never stepped before. I hope you become as excited as I am about this exercise programme and find that it makes a contribution towards a contented, active, positive and healthy lifestyle.

I wish you happy and successful stepping!

CHAPTER 2

Why Step?

What are the benefits of step aerobics? These are the main ones:

- It's a complete and balanced fitness programme in itself.
- You will improve your cardiovascular fitness, which will help to promote a healthy heart and lungs.
- You will efficiently burn calories and some of these calories may come from stores of body fat.
- You will firm and tone your hips, thighs and upper body.
- If you follow the whole of the programme you will tighten your abdominals and strengthen your back.

Stepping is an extremely efficient way of burning calories because it is a whole-body exercise involving large muscle groups in a rhythmic and dynamic action. The limited research available indicates that stepping is a more effective way of burning calories than most other forms of aerobic dance. However, it is difficult to be precise about exactly how many calories you will burn per step workout as there are so many variables involved. Metabolic rate, over-all body weight and efficiency of the stepping action all vary amongst individuals, making it difficult to give an exact indication of how much body fat you can lose in a step workout without using laboratory conditions for testing. However, in 1991 the American College of Sports Medicine gave some general guidelines which suggested that stepping can be equivalent to:

- jogging at between five and seven miles per hour
  or
- cycling at ten to fifteen miles per hour,
  in terms of the number of calories burned.

If you have ever run or cycled at these speeds I think you will agree with me when I say that it is quite challenging. Stepping for twenty or thirty minutes is nowhere near as arduous, and much more fun!

Early studies by Cisar and Kravitz (1991) on the effects of stepping on body-fat losses showed average fat losses of six pounds over a ten-week period of stepping three times a week. The subjects were both men and women of varying ages. Six pounds of fat over ten weeks (not six pounds of total body weight, which could include a large amount of water) is a considerable amount to lose and would indicate a steady and sensible weight loss that would be maintainable; in other words, not the sort that would go right back on again as soon as you went out for a celebration meal!

The step programme involves the use of all the major leg muscles, which is a great time saver in your daily workout. In most exercise programmes you complete the aerobic-exercise section, which conditions your cardio-vascular system and helps to burn calories, and then you need to get on to a mat on the floor and complete your conditioning exercises for legs and abdominals. This procedure can be lengthy, and de-motivating. With the step programme you can kill two birds with one stone by working your heart and lungs and, at the same time, improving the strength and tone of your leg and buttock muscles. Let's face it – you're far more likely to be able to devote thirty minutes three times a week to your exercise programme than twice this amount.

Note that the improvements you will get to the shape of your legs will mean tighter, firmer muscles and a more attractive shape – not bulky muscles, for this is not a heavy-weight-training programme; your own body weight provides the resistance.

• *It employs simple but challenging movement patterns*

Step choreography does not have to be complicated to be stimulating and effective. The advanced routines should challenge you, but people seem to find them easier to manage than a lot of the more dance-inspired aerobic movements. If my husband can manage most of them, anyone can!

• *It's a low-impact workout.*

Stepping will not jar your joints as jogging and jumping can. If you take careful note of the tips in **Step Safely**, Chapter 4, you will protect your joints and prevent them from injury by strengthening the supporting muscles.

Other forms of low-impact aerobic exercise have often failed to provide the intensity that more advanced exercisers want. With the step programme you can monitor it to suit your own needs by changing the step height or the speed of the music (advice included in **Step Safely**) and still keep your body free from injury.

• *It saves space when you exercise at home.*

How many times have you turned down exercise books or videos because you couldn't manage to fit all of the travelling movements into your lounge? All you need for this step programme is space to walk around the step, which should be feasible in most average-sized rooms.

The sudden emergence of step aerobics often leads people to believe that stepping up and down on to a bench or box is a relatively new way of getting fit. After all, it's only the past two or three years that have seen the advent of step classes and step videos. However, as far back as the 1960s, levels of aerobic fitness were being assessed by step tests; i.e., stepping up and down on to a wooden box or school-style bench for a set period of time. These tests are still offered in some health clubs today and are used to:

- assess suitability to begin an exercise programme; and,
- provide a yardstick upon which to measure fitness progress.

Any of the step tests on the market provide a good general indication of how fit you are cardiovascularly, but in those very early days of aerobic exercise they were never intended as an exercise programme in themselves. Certainly nobody in their wildest dreams would have imagined the styles and varieties of choreography available to 'steppers' now! It was all just 'up, down, up, down – plod plod, plod plod'!

I can remember exercising on a long wooden bench with a whole crowd of kids when I was at school. The noise of the 'up up, down down' really seemed to create a team spirit among us – a sense of achievement that we could actually keep in time with each other! The drumbeat-like thump was reassuring in a way. Children obviously still feel this way, as my children's step classes are tremendously popular. In fact, you may find that your teenage son or daughter will pinch your step and *Dyna-Step Challenge* to complete the programme themselves!

Remember though, that there are special considerations for children when exercising and I mention these towards the end of the book (see pages 210–212).

So, how did step aerobics as we see it now originate? Three or four years ago an experienced American exercise teacher, Gin Miller, had to stop teaching due to a serious knee injury. On the advice of a physiotherapist she began performing step exercises three times a day and found that it dramatically improved all aspects of her fitness, as well as strengthening her knee. As she recovered she gradually incorporated steps into some of her classes and was overwhelmed by the response from both men and women. Thus, step aerobics was born!

If you talk to people who regularly participate in step aerobics, either in a class or at home, you will often find that they comment on the steady beat and rhythm of stepping and that they enjoy the exercise because they know what's expected of them.

You just have to get on and off the step, which is far easier for many people than executing movement combinations in a more traditional aerobic manner. Consequently, stepping appeals to a wide variety of ages and fitness abilities. They include both men and women who vary in fitness background; for example, in my step classes at the moment I have a county rugby player, a national triathlete and, in contrast, some participants who have had no exercise experience whatsoever – some of whom have led very sedentary lives. The appeal of stepping is tremendous and we are at last seeing more men participating in aerobic classes.

Step aerobics doesn't have the 'dancy' image that some forms of aerobic exercise have. The programme also offers the option of using handweights to develop upper-body strength, which appeals to the physically fit and active, or those who are looking for a real challenge. Stepping can be very simply co-ordinated and

demanding enough to offer some real fitness benefits –
hence it's appeal to everyone!

WHICH STEP?

The two step challenges can be performed on almost any
step and, if you are thinking of purchasing a step other
than the Dyna-Step, consider the following pointers:

The Material

There are various types of polypropylene and fibreglass
steps on the market. In fact, it's easy to be confused by
the range of materials on offer, with terminology such as
'high molecular' and 'high density' appearing on all of
the literature.

I suggest you just try the step yourself – the material
should be durable and yet have some 'give' in it. If there
is no play at all in the material your footfalls will not be
softened and joint problems could eventually occur;
also, the step is more likely to crack after heavy usage.

The Platform

Some steps have a mat or other non-skid material on
their platforms. This can be useful, but check to see that
the matting is firmly attached and is made of strong rubber that will not 'bubble' or rip and cause accidents.

The Base

Look at the base of the step. If you are going to place
your step on a shiny floor surface (i.e., polished wood,
linoleum, tiles) then make sure the step can get a firm
grip on the floor. The Dyna-Step, for example, has rubber pads fixed on its base, which works very well. Other
steps have rubber feet or can be entirely rubber based. If
your step has rubber feet or attachments, are they

attached firmly or are you forever going to be finding yours under the sofa?

Size of Platform

The larger the platform the more intensity you can build into your travelling steps. However, space may be a problem so, depending on your storage situation, make sure that the width is enough to place your whole foot comfortably on, ideally at least fourteen inches, and the length is comfortable when performing travelling steps.

Step Height

Steps are either in a simple box format and are only one height, or they have some method involving building blocks or feet that make them height adjustable. The simple box is the least expensive but doesn't enable you to progress through your step programme gradually, as a high step may be too ambitious to start with but may be necessary as the weeks go by. If you decide to invest in a height adjustable step to give you more flexibility consider the following:

- How does the height mechanism work? Are there any clips snapping the legs or blocks into place that look as if they could break?
- Is the step totally secure at all heights? Generally speaking, the simpler the design the better as there is less to go wrong!

If you are still unsure I suggest that you go to your local sports retailer and have a chat about any steps they may have for sale. Try them for comfort and remember it's not always the most expensive that's the best. There are also companies that have steps for hire, so you could try a step programme on one before you commit yourself to purchasing.

Whichever step you choose to buy, it will be suitable for this exercise programme. And if you are still undecided I can thoroughly recommend the Dyna-Step!

Step aerobics is the latest fitness craze to sweep the country – but is it just a craze? Judging by the results my clients have achieved I don't think so. Stepping is definitely here to stay so why not begin the Dyna-Step Challenge right away and benefit from a firmer and healthier body, and enjoy yourself while achieving it!

CHAPTER 3
About the Challenge

The step programme that you are about to follow has been designed to be flexible enough for a wide range of abilities and ages. It is separated into four sections, which can be adapted to suit your daily schedule.

- _Warming Up_. This section takes approximately eight minutes.
- _New Stepper's Challenge_. Approximately fifteen minutes.
- _Advanced Dyna-Step Challenge_. Approximately twenty-five minutes.
- _Tight Tums and Healthy Backs_. Approximately five minutes.
- _Cooling Down_. Approximately three minutes.

The programme is flexible and your choice of sections will depend on the time (and energy) that you have available. You must always warm up and cool down before any exercise, and the step programme is no exception, but you can opt to do the step section one day, and the optional tum and back exercises on alternate days. This would give you a short workout on six days of the week.

For example: _Day One_
Warm Up
Step Section
Cool Down

Day Two
Warm Up
Tums and Backs
Cool Down

This pattern would be repeated on Days Three, Four, Five, Six and Day Seven would be a rest day.

Alternatively you can go through the whole programme on three days of every week giving yourself a rest day between each workout. If you perform the whole programme in one go it should take about thirty minutes if you are a new stepper, and about forty minutes for the advanced programme.

BEGINNER OR ADVANCED STEPPER?

The secret of success in any exercise programme is to begin at a low level and build up gradually – like going through the gears of your car. If you try to start in fifth gear your car will rebel and give out on you. Your body would probably react in the same way if you attempted to take on an advanced programme before you are ready for it. In other words, don't run before you can walk or you may become demoralized and give up.

I mention this because there may be some of you who feel that, as you are reasonably physically fit and have exercised before, you could begin straightaway with the Advanced Dyna-Step Challenge. This may be unwise because if stepping is new to you you'll have to get used to the new movement combinations and this may frustrate you if you fail to co-ordinate the steps in the advanced challenge.

The general rules should be:

• *New steppers*, whether experienced in other forms of exercise or not, start with the New Stepper's Challenge. You may find, if you are reasonably physically fit, that you can move up to the advanced workout within five or six sessions.

- *Experienced steppers*, you should be able to move straight into the Advanced Challenge providing that you are physically fit and exercise regularly.

However, if you are in any doubt, adopt the safest course of action and start at the beginning with the New Stepper's Challenge.

HOW CAN YOU ASSESS WHICH IS THE RIGHT LEVEL FOR YOU?

'Listen to your body' is a phrase often used when talking about appropriate levels or intensities of exercise. To judge how hard you are working by how you feel at the time of exercising may seem rather vague and unscientific. Studies have shown, however, that listening to your body can be quite an accurate assessment of the intensity of exercise.

You should be able to:

- Comfortably have a conversation with someone while stepping – in other words, you should not be breathless to the extent that speaking is difficult.
- Perform the movements smoothly and safely (see Chapter 4, **Step Safely**).
- You should feel no pain or discomfort.
- You may be red in the face but this is not a problem – it's just a sign that you are getting warm and your body is disposing of heat via your skin. I go beetroot red when I am stepping!

You need to work within your limits and yet work hard enough to attain some benefits. You may like to use the perceived scale of exertion, on the following page. This scale was devised in the 1970s by Borg, an exercise physiologist, and has proved to be reasonably accurate. We all seem to have an inbuilt sense of what is and what isn't comfortable in many situations, perhaps not just during exercise.

Perceived Exertion Scale

Rating	Description
6	Very, very light
9	Very light
10	
11	Fairly light
12	
13	Somewhat hard
14	
15	Hard
16	
17	Very hard
18	
19	Very, very hard

To achieve a 'training effect' – i.e., to benefit from the exercise and be able to progress – you should be working at somewhere between levels twelve and fifteen, once you are into your stepping phase. This is a purely subjective way of assessing effort levels, but it is convenient for you to use while stepping, is not disruptive and, after all, you should be able to judge whether or not you are comfortable – you know your own body!

A more accurate way of assessing the intensity of your workout is to measure your heart rate. The more blood that is pumped around your body to your muscles the faster your heart has to beat. Measuring your heart rate while participating in a step routine would be impossible and could affect your balance! If you wish to measure your heart rate you would have to check your pulse at the end of the stepping routine, which means that you will have cooled down and your heart rate will probably be lower than it was when you were energetically stepping. Bear this in mind when you calculate a heart-rate score, particularly if it is below your target range.

Personal Target Heart Rate

If you do decide to measure your heart rate in order to judge whether you are working at an appropriate level, use the following formula:

> 220 minus your age;
>
> multiplied by 60%; and
>
> multiplied by 85%.

For example, if you are thirty-five, your target heart rates are:

> 220 minus 35 equals 185;
>
> 185 multiplied by 60% equals 111; and
>
> 185 multiplied by 85% equals 157.

Therefore, a thirty-five-year-old stepper would need to work at a heart rate of between 111 and 157 for the exercise to be both safe and effective.

If this all seems quite complicated, stick to the perceived exertion method; i.e., how you feel at the time of exercising. If you wish to measure your heart rate, practise locating your radial artery, which lies along the thumb side of your wrist about two inches above the base of your thumb. Use your two forefingers to count the beats. Don't use your thumb, which has a clear pulse of its own which may confuse you. Count for ten seconds and multiply your score by six to give you the beats per minute.

As you find your workout becoming easier, and maybe your heart rate lowering and not reaching your target, there are various ways of upping the intensity of the programme, which we will discuss in later chapters. These include increasing the height of your step, adding more power moves – with or without the use of handweights – and speeding up the rate of stepping a little. You need to adhere to strict safety guidelines when adopting any of these methods of increasing intensity, which leads me nicely into the next chapter!

CHAPTER 4
Step Safely

It is essential that you read these guidelines before you begin the exercises in either of the step challenges.

Footwear/Clothing

Repeated stepping up and down on to a bench or block without training shoes could be injurious. There are training shoes on the market specifically designed for stepping which are light and flexible, and yet supportive and machine washable! However, they tend to be expensive and, bearing in mind their unsuitability for outdoor activities and high-impact aerobic classes, you may find it more economical to invest in a 'cross trainer' or general-purpose shoe. The range of training shoes available is extensive – talk to your local sports retailer about a supportive shoe that is flexible enough to allow for foot movement, and is comfortable.

Clothing needs to be light, comfortable and non-restrictive. You may find that you sweat more while stepping than during other forms of exercise. It is important, therefore, to be suitably dressed – tight jeans will be inappropriate!

Many experienced steppers find that they become exceptionally thirsty during and after their step workout, so you need to prepare yourself for this. Make sure that you start the step section well hydrated by drinking a glass of water, and then continue to drink small amounts in stages during the workout and again when you have finished. If you really do sweat excessively make sure that the top of your step does not become slippery – have a towel handy to mop yourself and your step down! The consistent use of the major leg and buttock muscles means that you are working very hard, even though it may not feel excessively demanding. Take short breaks during the step routine to drink water or mop yourself up, but try to keep your legs moving rather than standing completely still or you could become dizzy. I advise you not to drink and step at the same time!

Step Height

Studies have shown that the most significant way of altering the intensity of your step routine is by adjusting the height of your step. If you have purchased a step that is not height adjustable you are obviously restricted to working at this one level and will have to adjust the intensity of the workout to suit you by a change in music speed, as mentioned below, or an increase in the size of your movements, as mentioned in each step routine.

If you are able to adjust the height of your step I would advise you to follow these guidelines:

• *New steppers*. Begin on the lowest level possible. This will be five inches if you have the Dyna-Step or maybe four or six inches with other steps. Increase the height of your step gradually as you begin to feel comfortable with the step movements and feel that the intensity of the exercise is manageable; in other words, you can hold a conversation while you are stepping rather than being completely out of breath. An eight-inch-high step will provide an effective workout for experienced steppers – any higher than this and you may compromise the technique of the exercise (i.e., good form, posture and alignment may become difficult to maintain and injuries could result). Often I see ambitious steppers attempting to work on a ten- or even twelve-inch step. As fatigue begins to set in they look as though they are trying to climb Mount Everest and literally have to throw themselves into the upward step movement!

• *Experienced steppers*. Depending on the length of time you have been stepping and the frequency (i.e., once, twice or three times a week), you need to select either a six- or eight-inch-high step. If you begin with the New Stepper's Challenge in order to familiarize yourself with the sequences, an eight-inch step would be appropriate. If you decide to 'go for it' and start with the Advanced Dyna-Step Challenge, begin with a five- or six-inch step if you can, and then when you feel comfortable with the routines increase the height.

Music Speed

The faster you step the harder your heart has to work to supply your muscles with oxygen. Music speed can have quite a significant effect on intensity, therefore you need to choose wisely. You can't really complete a step workout without music because when you have no beat to follow, steps can speed up or slow down according to how you feel at the time, which will make the level at which you work vary from session to session. If you have no beat to follow, the steps will not flow and your workout will become stilted. And then there are the motivational advantages of working to music and the atmosphere it can create.

You can also sing along to your favourite music and forget the fact that you are working so hard! Therefore it is worth spending some time selecting your music. Although faster stepping will make you work harder, there is a limit as to how fast you can safely step and still maintain good posture and alignment. Sprint stepping for fifteen or twenty-five minutes would also be extremely tiring!

The speed of your music should be somewhere between 118 and 124 beats per minute (or bpm, as stated on some record labels). This gives you quite a wide choice, as masses of popular chart music seems to fall into this range. Some of the 'oldies' from the 1960s and 1970s are much faster than this. Start listening to music on the radio and try stepping to it – this is the best way to check which speed is most comfortable. If it feels OK, use your watch or clock to check that the speed is in the correct range. Time your music by counting the strong drumbeat over fifteen seconds and then multiply by four to give you the total beats per minute. Some records have already done this for you and the speed is noted on the cassette or record label.

New steppers need to work at between 118 and 120 beats per minute, and stay at this speed until the programme feels comfortable and you are competent at performing the steps. You may feel content to stay at this speed indefinitely and to increase the intensity by raising your step height.

I would advise against increasing the speed of your music and the step height all in the same week! All exercise should be gradually progressive – as smoothly progressed as driving up through the gears when driving a car!

Use of Handweights

Studies are unclear, at the moment, as to whether the use of handweights during the step sequences significantly increases intensity. Arm movements with hand-held weights need to be slow, controlled, short-lever movements which are indicated in the step challenge section. If you are very physically fit, like Steve who is the model for the advanced challenge, you should be able to maintain good-quality stepping with one- to two-pound handweights. If you opt to use weights, avoid fast snappy arm movements and don't hold your arms above your head for long periods of time.

The arm choreography in both step routines is appropriate for use with handweights but, if you feel unsure and are still not completely confident with the arm patterns, rather than use handweights which may or may not make your workout harder, use bigger leg movements, deeper bends on the squats and lunges, and maybe add some jumps into your steps where suggested.

Steve is using two one-pound handweights on the Advanced Dyna-Step Challenge – but only on some selected arm movements. He feels that, rather than making his heart and lungs work harder, the weights help to maintain his upper-body strength and he will not need to work this area after the step sequences, therefore saving him valuable time. Steve is, however, extremely fit, and he is able to maintain good technique throughout the routine when he is holding the weights.

EXERCISE TECHNIQUE

It is vitally important that you practise the technique of stepping before you launch yourself into either of the step challenges. I realize that it may be difficult for you to check your body positions in a mirror – the bathroom cabinet mirror will be far too small! Get a friend/relative to look at the photographs and tell you whether you are doing it right. Start as you mean to go on – performing the moves correctly and therefore getting the best out of your workout. It may all seem a bit of a bore having to go through all this when you want to get going on your step but, do it now and those good habits will become ingrained into your routines.

Good Posture

- Shoulders back and relaxed;
- tummy pulled in;
- pelvis tilted forward; and
- knees slightly bent,

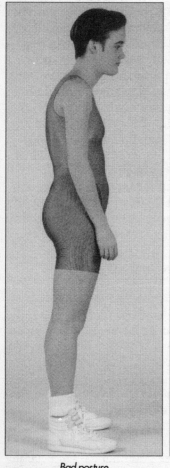

Bad posture

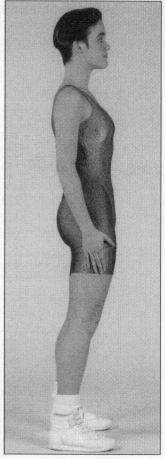

Good posture

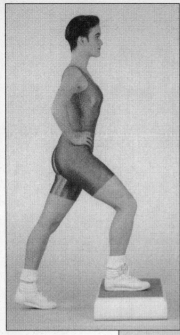

Look at how you can change your shape in seconds, just by adopting a good postural position! Try to keep reminding yourself of this position throughout your step workout. As you step up there should be a diagonal line from your heel to your head. In other words your whole body should lean from your heel – not from the middle of your body as illustrated.

Correct step-up

Incorrect step-up

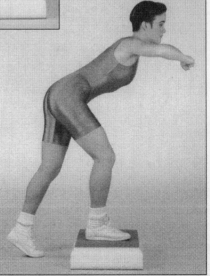

Once on top of the step and performing Knee Lifts or Side Leg Raises, etc., keep your back straight and tum pulled in rather than arch your back, throwing your shoulders backwards as shown.

Correct—straight back

Incorrect—arched back

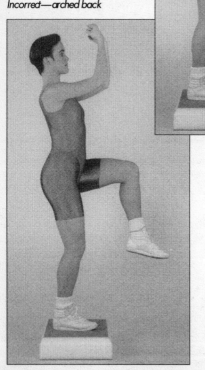

Foot Placement

• Step into the centre of your platform.

• Place your whole foot on the step – you may have to look down at your step every now and then to make sure that your heel or toe is not hanging over the edge of the step. If this happens repeatedly you may experience some lower-leg soreness, and you are also more likely to overbalance.

• When pushing up from the floor, lift the heel then ball and toe of the foot.

• When stepping down, which is the movement which seems to cause the most lower-leg soreness because it can be uncontrolled, reverse the action to the ball of the foot first and then the heel. Keep close to your step as you step down.

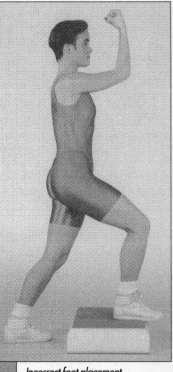

Incorrect foot placement

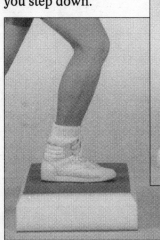

Correct foot placement

Knee Flexion

• On stepping up on to your step, make sure that your knee never bends at less than a right (ninety-degree) angle or you may damage the ligaments which act as support in the knee joint. You are more likely to hyper-flex (bend to excess) your knee if your step is too high for your leg length or fitness ability.

I find that with the schoolchildren that I teach many of them work on a very low step because they have shorter legs than adults and not necessarily because they are unfit.

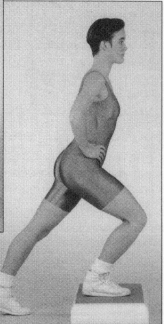

Correct knee flexion

Incorrect knee flexion

Throughout the exercises make sure that your knees are very slightly bent rather than completely locked. This will protect your spine and your knees.

Quality of Movement

Try to perform the exercises as smoothly as possible and avoid jerky and uncontrolled movements. Practise some of the steps before you put them to music so that it gives you the chance to rehearse them at slow tempo.

Other safety points to note are:

• Always familiarize yourself with the footwork before you attempt to add the arm movements. Your brain may not be able to cope with more than one concept at a time!
• Stay close to your step and look down at it every now and then to check your foot placement. If you step too far away from your step you may miss it completely when you become involved in a more complicated sequence, or enthusiasm takes over once you are in full flow.
• You will notice that none of the movements ask you to stand with your back to the step and to step up on to the platform backwards; this could be dangerous.
• Never step forward off the step – the routines don't ask you to do this either; this has been shown to exert a force on the knee which can be up to six times your body weight!

Step Injuries

You are no more likely to incur injuries through stepping than in any other exercise programme providing that you follow the safety guidelines. Over-training could cause an injury, so if you become as hooked on stepping as I am you would be wise to remind yourself that three step sessions per week is extremely effective in terms of calorie-burning and muscle-toning. More than this could well lead to over-use injuries, such as knee, lower-leg and back problems. Again, this would be true of any physical activity that is performed to excess.

The step sequences in both the New Stepper's and the Advanced Dyna-Step Challenges have been designed with safety and injury prevention primarily in mind. Providing that you follow the teaching instructions and guidelines you are sure to have a safe, effective and enjoyable workout!

Before you do, ask yourself if there are any reasons why you may not be suited to step exercises.

- Have you any history of heart disease?
- Do you suffer from high blood pressure?
- Do you have any joint problems?
- Are you pregnant or have you recently had a baby? (See Chapter 10, **Special Steppers**)
- Are you taking any medication that may preclude exercise?

If the answer is yes to any of these questions then please contact your doctor to discuss the suitability of this exercise programme for you.

Without further ado, let's get on to the warm-up!

CHAPTER 5
Warming Up

I realize how tempting it is to go straight into your step challenge without warming up, to save time. Life can be hectic and saving ten minutes or so can seem attractive. However, to miss out on warming up will be false economy. Your body will not be thoroughly mentally and physically prepared for the step exercises and you may injure your joints or muscles. Remember the analogy of the car going through its gears? We can once again apply this to our bodies when exercising. Physical activity should start at a very low level, with non-strenuous movements, and then gradually build up to larger and more intensive movements. Our heart, lungs, joints and muscles will then be allowed to adapt to the increased demands gradually and safely. Rush straight into your workout without careful warming up and you are at risk of straining or spraining muscles, ligaments and tendons. An investment of your time spent on this section will be worthwhile.

As your level of physical fitness increases you may find that it will take less time for your body to become warm. This is because, physiologically, your body is responding more quickly to the exercises as it has become used to warming up. For a new exerciser the warm-up section may take ten to twelve minutes or more, whereas an advanced exerciser may only need seven or eight minutes (this would be a minimum and may possibly have to be increased in cold weather when your body will take longer to warm up). You need to adapt the repetitions on the warm-up exercises to suit your individual level.

You may feel that it would be more fun to warm up to music. You could use the same speed of music as suggested for your step routine or even slightly faster. Remember, though, you should be able to complete all of the movements comfortably at the speed you have chosen.

Safety points:

- You must feel warm before you go into the stretches. Stretching cold muscles can lead to muscle strains and tears.
- Adjust the length of the warm-up to suit you; continue marching or punching across with your arms until you feel warm, motivated and ready to go.
- Have your step ready to use as a support in the stretches at the end of the warm-up.
- Clear a good space around the step.
- Have some drinking water and a towel handy.
- Switch off the telephone.

Off you go!

Shoulder Lifts

- Stand with your feet slightly more than hip distance apart.

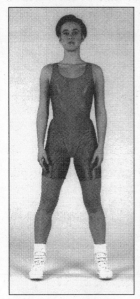

- Knees should be relaxed and not locked.
- Tummy pulled in and back straight.
- Breathe normally.
- Squeeze your shoulders up to your ears and relax back down.
- Repeat this 8 times.

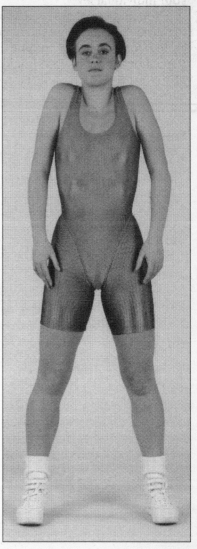

Shoulder Rolls

- Standing in the
  same position as the
  Shoulder Lifts.

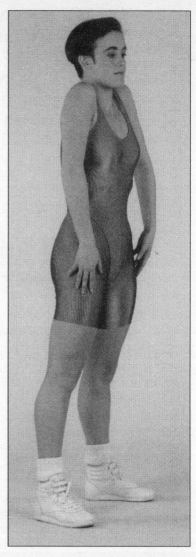

- Roll your shoulders gently round by squeezing them up to your ears, pulling them backwards, down and then forwards to make a circle.
- Repeat 8 times.

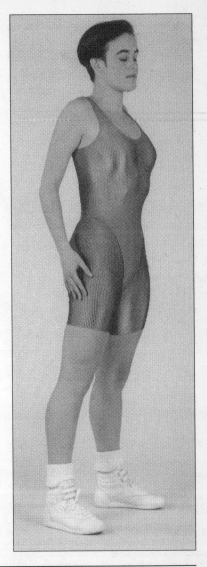

Arm Circles

- Keeping your elbows bent, circle your arms and shoulders smoothly around.
- Repeat 8 times.

Perform the Shoulder Lifts, Shoulder Rolls and Arm Circles again to ensure that your shoulder area is thoroughly warmed up.

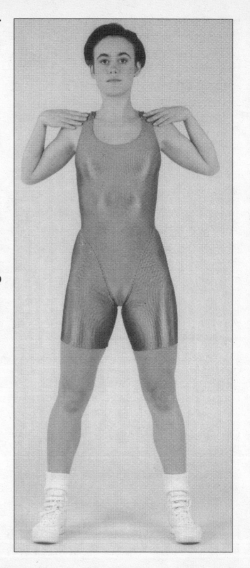

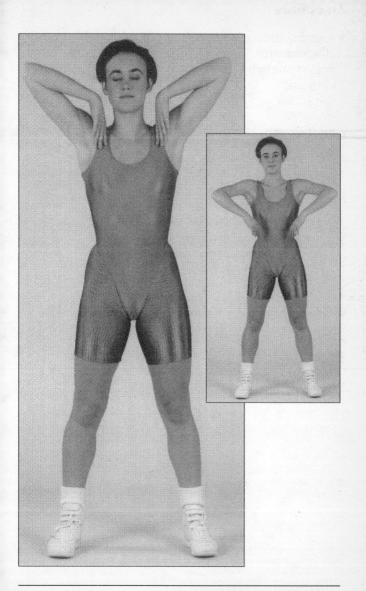

Side Bends

- Again standing in the correct postural position as described for Shoulder Lifts. It is particularly important that the knees are not locked in this exercise.

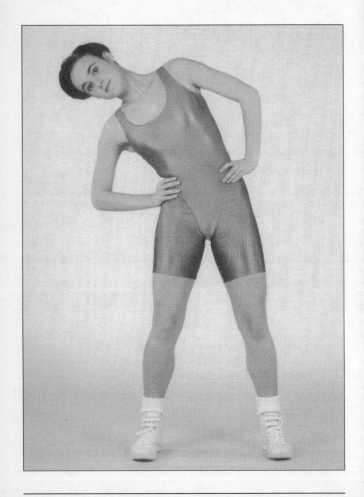

- Bend from your waist directly to the side.
- Try not to lean either forward or back – imagine you are sandwiched between two panes of glass!
- Repeat 8 Side Bends to the right, and 8 to the left.

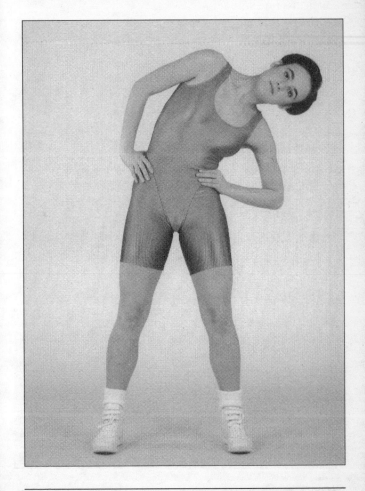

Trunk Twists

- In the same position as for Side Bends.
- Twist from your waist to one side.
- Take your head with you in the twist so that you are looking over your shoulder.
- Keep your hips, knees and feet facing forward.
- Only twist round as far as you can comfortably.
- Do 8 twists right and 8 left.

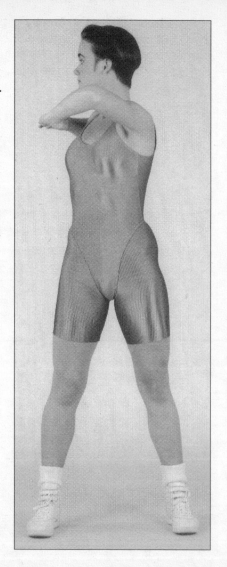

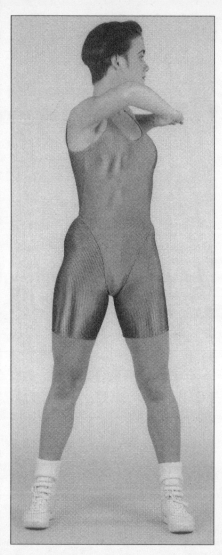

Repeat Side
Bends and Trunk
Twists through
again to warm up
the spine.

Hip Swings

- Keeping your knees slightly bent, swing your hips from side to side. Keep the movements smooth and controlled.
- Repeat 16 times.

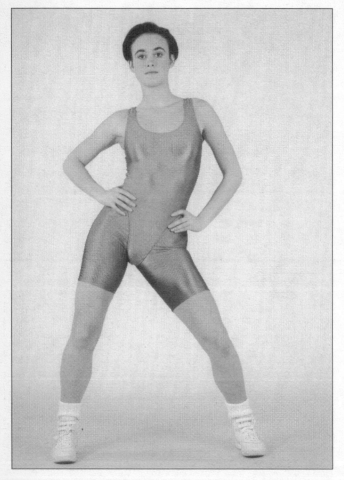

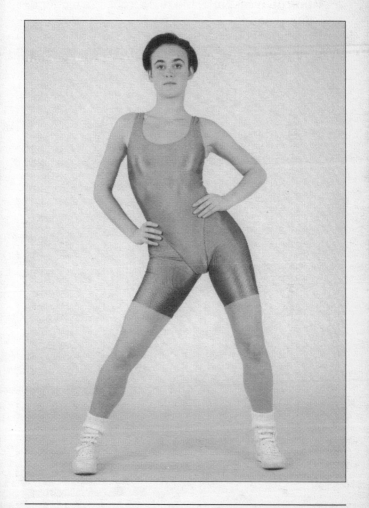

Ankle Circles

- Circle one foot around to loosen and warm your ankle.
- Keep the knee of your standing leg bent.
- If you need support, hold on to a chair or a door or wall.
- Do 4 circles on each foot and repeat.

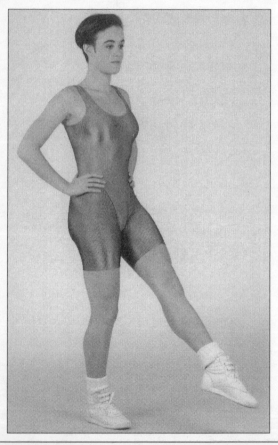

Marching

- When you march, place the ball of your foot down first and then your heel to follow.
- Make your marching progressively more energetic by using higher leg movements and swinging your arms.
- Do this for a minute or so until you start to feel warmer. If you have the space, walk around your room, or around the garden if it's a sunny day.

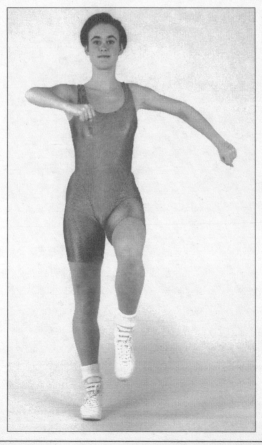

Side-to-Side Sway

- Keeping your posture upright and tall, shift your weight from one foot to the other.
- The more you bend your knees, the more energetic the movement will become.
- Repeat 8 times.

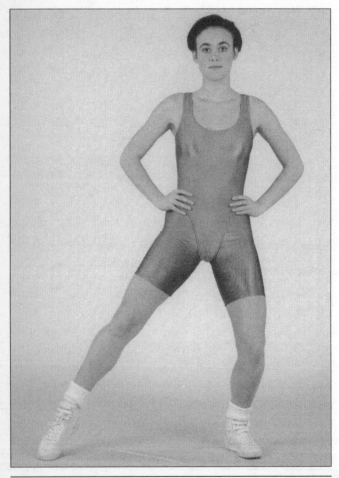

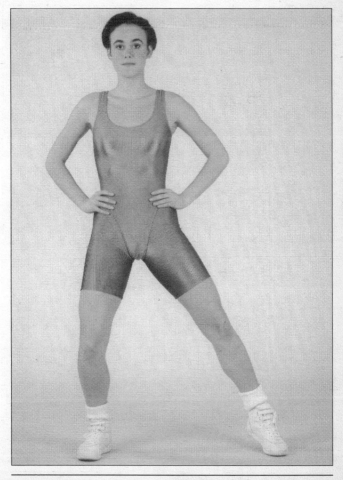

Punch Across

- Keep going with the Side-to-Side Sway and punch your arms across your body alternatively.
- Repeat 8 punches to each side.

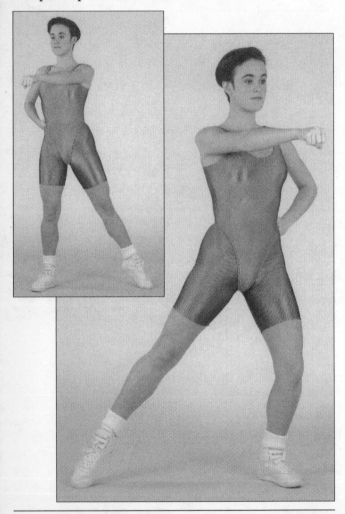

Punch Up

- The arms now punch up alternately, still keeping the feet in the Side-to-Side Sway.
- Repeat 8 punches with each arm.

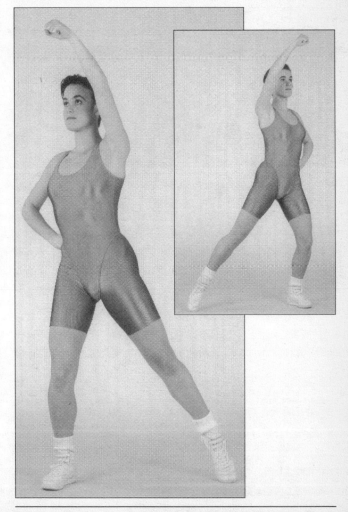

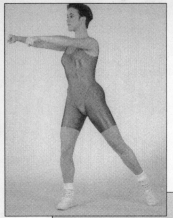

Now repeat the Punch Across and Punch Up movements, but using both arms at the same time.

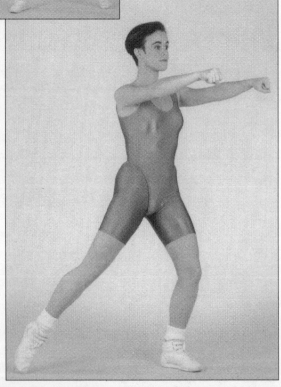

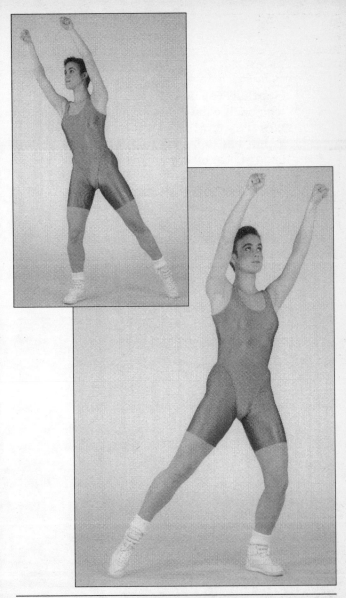

Hopefully you now feel that your body temperature has increased and you are nice and warm. Perhaps your sweat- or T-shirt has to be removed, which is a good indication of your increased body temperature. You should be ready to stretch out your major muscle groups, but if you don't feel warm yet then repeat the sections from Marching through to the Punch sequence again.

Have your step available to help you to perform these stretches.

Calf Stretch

- Place one foot on your step.
- Extend the other leg behind you.
- Both feet should be facing forwards (check the foot on the floor to make sure your toe is not turned out).
- The knee of the leg on the step should be bent.
- Body weight should be slightly forward.
- Place your hands on your thighs for support.
- You should feel the stretch in the back of your lower leg (calf).
- Hold for approximately 8 seconds.

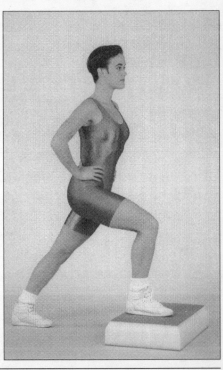

Hip Flexor Stretch

From the Calf Stretch position:
- Dip the knee of the back leg.
- Push the hip forward so that you feel a stretch across the top front thigh and over your hip.
- Hold on to the step for balance, if necessary.
- Hold the stretch for approximately 8 seconds.

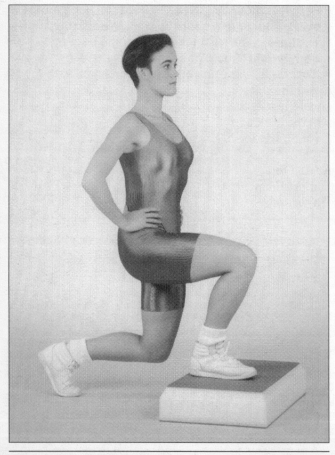

Back of Thigh – Hamstring

From the Hip Flexor Stretch above:
- Bend the back leg and straighten the leg that is on the step.
- To increase the stretch, lean forward from your hips – but only as far as is comfortable. Some people are extremely stiff and inflexible in this area, so take care.
- Rest your hands on your thighs to support your body weight and not on your knee joints, which can be vulnerable.
- Hold for 8 seconds.

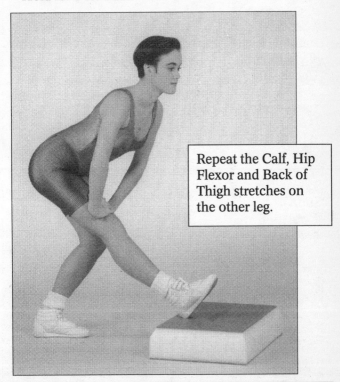

Repeat the Calf, Hip Flexor and Back of Thigh stretches on the other leg.

Front Thigh – Quadriceps

- Stand away from your step.
- Lift one leg behind you by taking the middle part of your foot in one hand. If you can't quite reach that far, hold the heel of your shoe.
- Keep the standing leg slightly bent.
- Check your posture – make sure your back is not arched. If balance is a problem hold on to a chair or wall for support.
- Hold for 8 seconds.

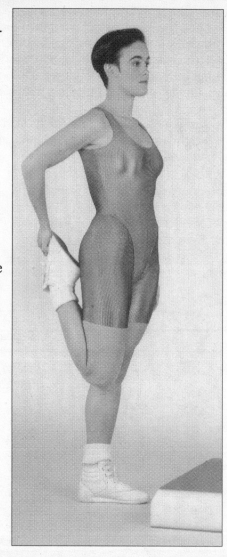

Underarm – Tricep

- Bend one arm and slide your hand down your back near your shoulder blades.
- Gently push with your other hand to increase the stretch (apply pressure to the fleshy part of your arm rather than near to your elbow).
- Hold for 8 seconds and then repeat on the other arm.

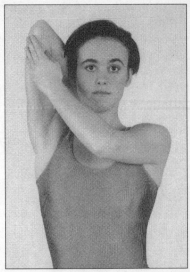

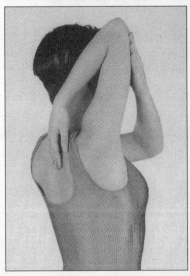

Chest – Pectoral

- Link your hands behind your back and pull your shoulder blades together.
- You should feel a stretch across your chest.
- Remember to maintain good posture throughout the stretch.
- Hold for approximately 8 seconds.

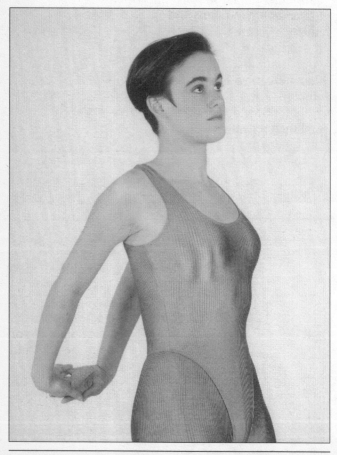

Deep Breath

- Take a deep breath in and reach your arms above you.
- Feel your chest expand and your lungs inflate.
- Breathe out and lower your arms.
- Shake out your arms and legs.

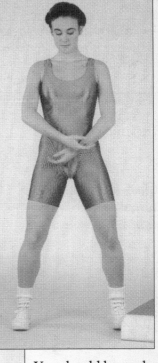

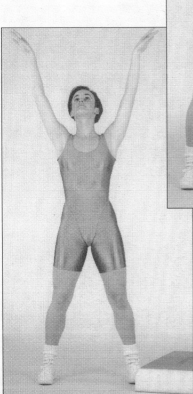

You should be ready to go either to the New-Stepper's or Advanced Dyna-Step Challenge – or maybe the Tum and Back exercises if you are splitting up your workout as we discussed in Chapter 3.

CHAPTER 6

NewStepper s Challenge

Here are some exercise terms with which you need to become acquainted in order to understand clearly the step routines.

STEP ATTACK

These are the different positions from which you can 'attack' your step.

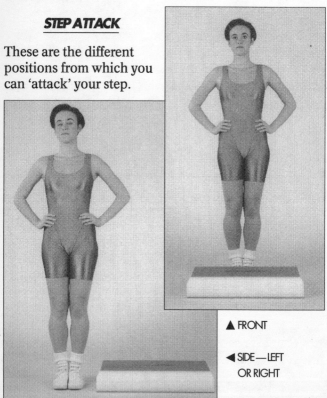

▲ FRONT

◄ SIDE—LEFT OR RIGHT

All of these terms will be used in the descriptions of the sequences.

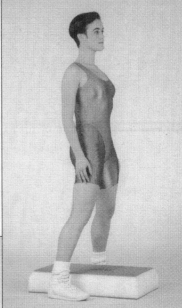

ASTRIDE ▶

▼ END

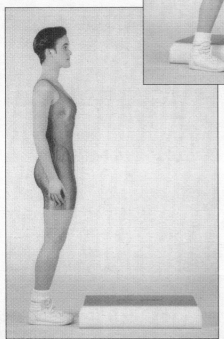

ON TOP ▶

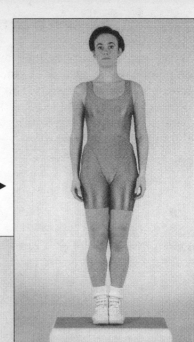

▼ DIAGONAL

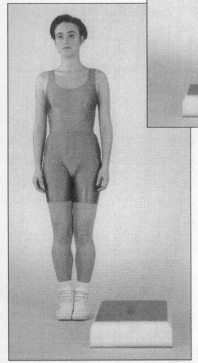

ARM EXERCISES

When you get to the stage where you are able to complete arm as well as leg movements, here are the names of the arm exercises that will be used in the sequences. Become familiar with the leg patterns first, because working arms and legs together can tend to throw you out of sequence.

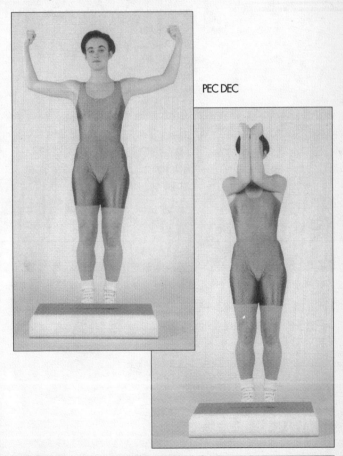

PEC DEC

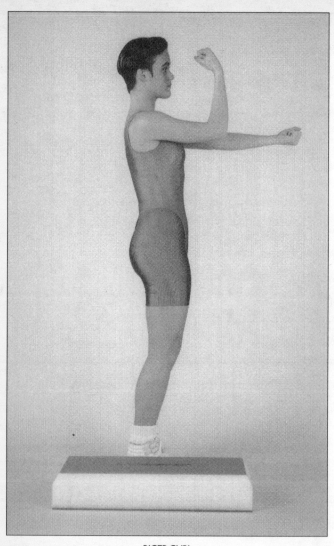

BICEP CURL

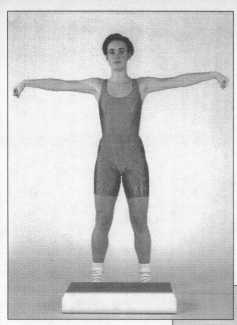

ELBOW KICK

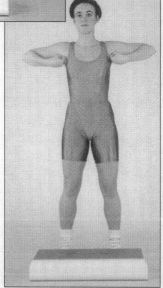

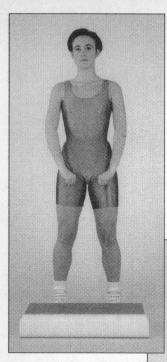

UPRIGHT ROW

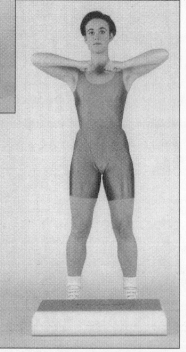

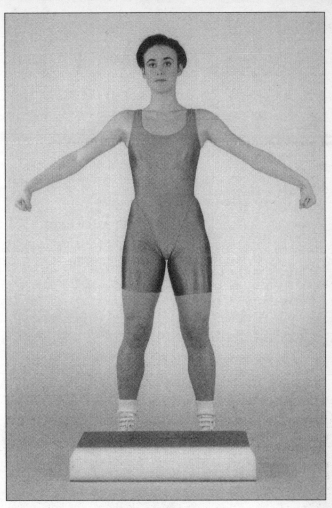

SHOULDER RAISE

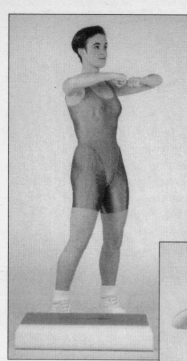

SHOULDER PULL-BACK

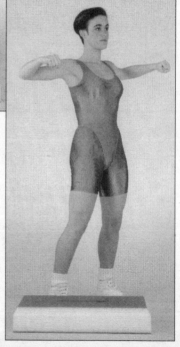

THE STEPS

Progress through this step routine will probably be slow and laborious at first, and you may wish to learn the steps without music, which will allow you to step at your own pace. You should not experience any pain or discomfort during the step challenge and you should not feel uncomfortably breathless. Persevere with the steps – they may seem complex at first, but once you get used to them they'll seem like second nature!

Well – here we go with the steps!

Three Marches and a Heel Dig

- This step will familiarize you with the height and position of your step.
- Safety points: Stay close to your step and remember the postural points made in Chapter 4, **Step Safely**.

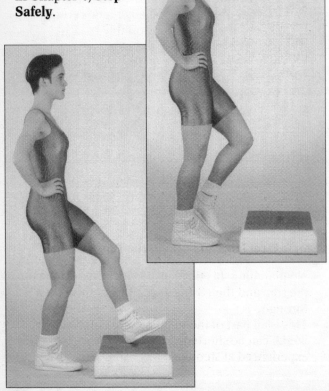

Three Marches and a Toe Tap

- Do the same sequence as opposite, only this time tap your toe on to the top of the step.
- Alternate the Heel Dig and Toe Tap combination for 8 counts each, and then repeat through twice more.

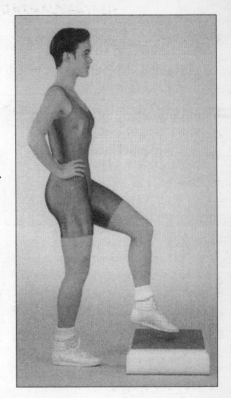

Single Heel Digs and Single Toe Taps

- No marching this time, just 8 Heel Digs on the top of the step and then 8 Toe Taps. Repeat this twice through.
- This is all part of the step familiarization routine which can be shortened when you become more experienced at stepping.

March on Top

- Your whole foot must be placed on the step when marching on top. This step will give you a feel for the width of the step.
- Safety points: Remember to keep your posture tall, knees slightly bent and tum tucked in.

March on the Floor

- Alternate the marches on the top of the step with the marches on the floor.
- Start with 8 marches on top and 8 marches on the floor.
- Gradually decrease this to 4 on top and 4 on the floor; then 2 on top and 2 on the floor.
- Repeat this a few times until you feel comfortable with the step height and width, and the speed of your music.

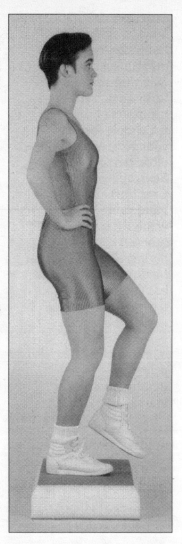

Simple Step – Right Lead

- Step up and down, always leading with the right leg.
- Safety points: Lean from your heel and not the middle of your body, as illustrated in **Step Safely**, Chapter 4.
- Place your whole foot centrally on the step.
- Land carefully back down on the floor by placing the ball of your foot, followed by your heel.
- Repeat this 8 times.

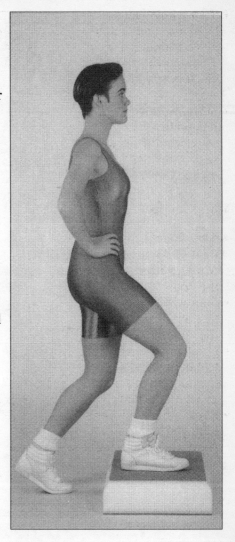

Simple Step – Left Lead

- Change so that your left leg is now leading first. To change lead leg you need to tap change (in this case after you step down with your right foot your left toe taps on the floor and comes straight back on to the step to lead).
- Repeat 8 times with the left leg.

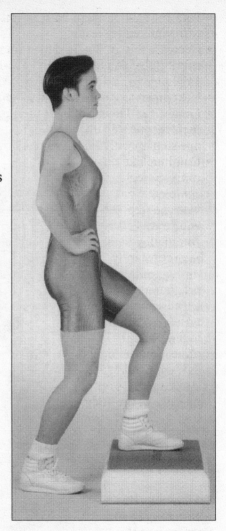

Tap-Down Change

- Perform 8 simple steps with a right-leg lead and 8 with your left leg leading.
- Decrease this gradually, depending on how comfortable you feel with the Tap-Down Change, to 4 right lead and 4 left lead.
- Next down to 2 right lead and 2 left lead.
- Finally, Tap-Down Change alternately so that you perform one step up with the right leg leading and one step up with the left leg leading.
- Continue like this until you feel completely happy with the step. We will be using this Alternating Lead Step constantly throughout the programme. This is because it would be unsafe to continue to lead with the same leg indefinitely as there would be constant stress on one side of the body.

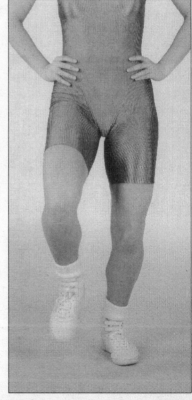

Maintaining this Alternating Lead Step, go into the following steps.

V-Step Combination

- Right-leg lead.

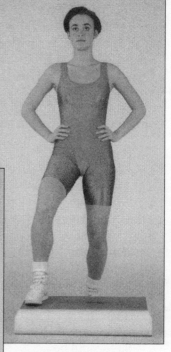

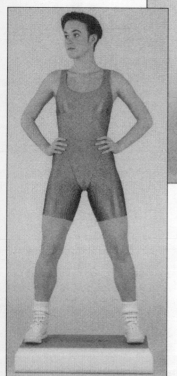

- On top, legs wide.

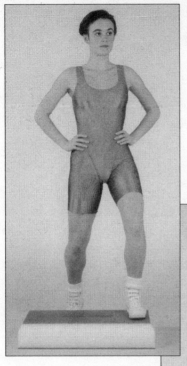

- Right leg returns to the floor.
- Lower down and tap change to lead with the left leg.

Perform 8 V-Steps and then 8 alternating Tap-Down steps with the feet stepping close together and not wide apart as in the V-Step. Continue with this combination of V-Steps and Alternating Simple Steps for 3 or 4 repeats.

The arm movements to go with this are:

- Shoulder Raises for the
  Simple Step and
  alternating Shoulder
  Pull-Backs for the V-
  Step; i.e., when the right
  leg steps up, the right
  arm goes up, the left arm
  extends when the left leg
  steps up and on the
  descent the shoulders
  pull back.

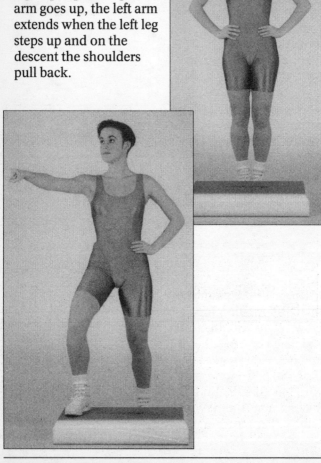

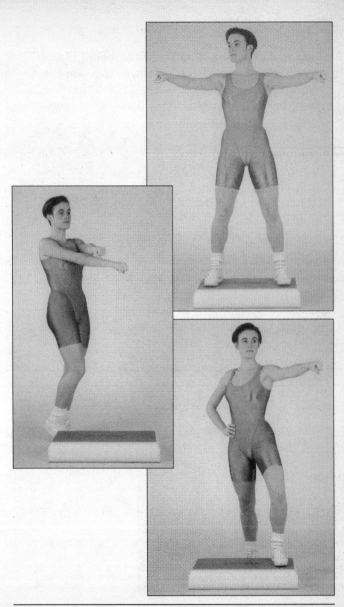

V-Step with Lunge

- Progress the V-Step now by turning your hips inwards as you finish the V-Step, so that you are making an arc or horseshoe shape with your body.
- Take the leg that taps down into a lunge behind you.

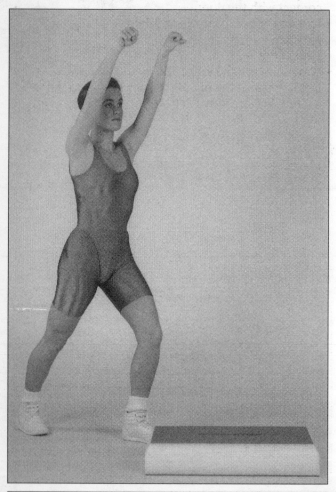

- The further you lunge behind the harder you have to start working.
- Safety points: Don't attempt to force your heel down on the lunge, only the ball of your foot needs to make contact with the floor.
- Extend your arms overhead when you lunge, if you are able.
- Repeat this movement 16 times.
- Now leave out the lunge and gradually bring your feet in towards the middle of your step from the wide V-Step. You are now back to the Alternating Lead Step.

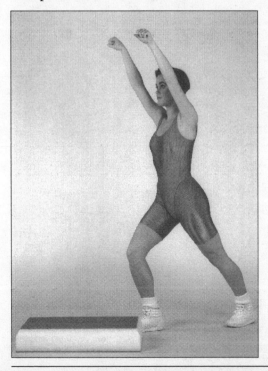

Knee Lift – Right-Leg Lead

- Step up with your right leg and lift your left leg into a Knee Lift.
- Now place the left leg straight back down on to the floor without it touching the step.

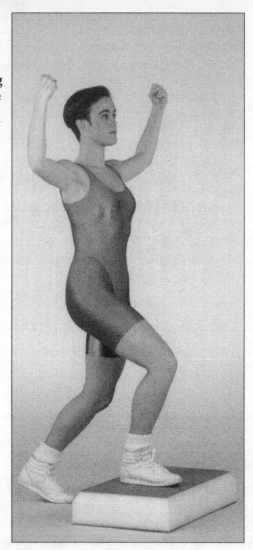

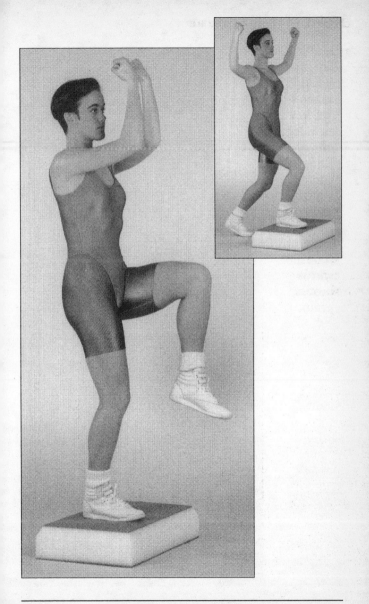

Knee Lift – Left-Leg Lead

- Your left leg taps down and lifts on to the step, and your right leg lifts up in a Knee Lift, going straight back to the floor to tap down and start the whole process again.

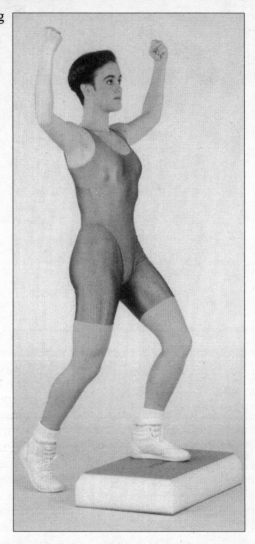

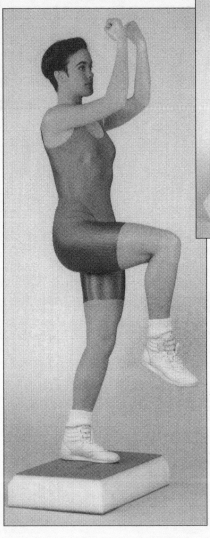
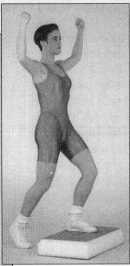

- Safety points:
  Keep your back
  straight as you
  lift your knee –
  don't be too
  ambitious and
  attempt to lift
  your knee too
  high.
- Repeat this
  movement until
  you are happy
  that you have
  mastered it.

Travelling Knee Lift – Right-Leg Lead

- Travel the Knee Lift across the length of your step by turning your hips; i.e., left hip towards the right end of the step and right hip towards the left end of the step.

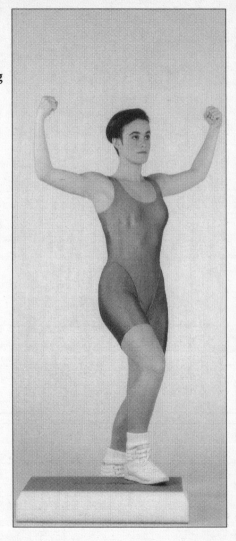

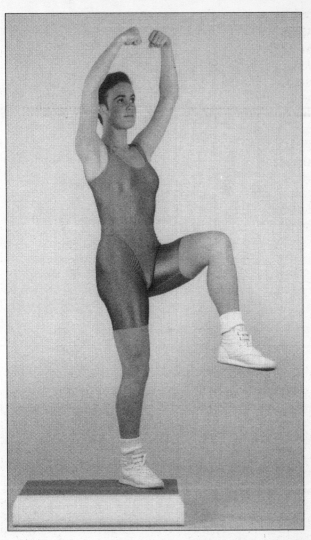

Step down and travel to:

Travelling Knee Lift – Left-Leg Lead

- Safety points are the same as for the basic Knee Lift without travelling.

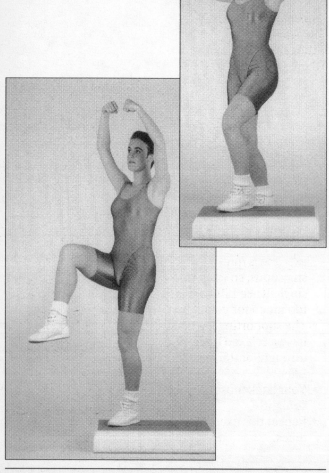

Bridging Arm Movement

- While you are standing behind the step and are about to travel to the other side, perform a Pec Dec arms movement.
- Repeat the Travelling Knee Lift 8 times to each side.

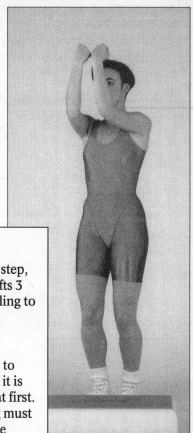

Repeaters

- At each end of the step, repeat the Knee Lifts 3 times before travelling to the other end.
- Safety points: This exercise is quite strenuous, so keep to single Knee Lifts if it is too much for you at first.
- The supporting leg must have a relaxed knee throughout the 3 Knee Lifts.
- Your back must be straight.
- Repeat this exercise 8 times.

Side Leg Squeeze

- Now substitute the Knee Lift with a Side Leg Squeeze as shown.
- Safety points: As you lift your leg out to the side, keep your body upright rather than leaning to one side. If you attempt to lift your leg too high you will

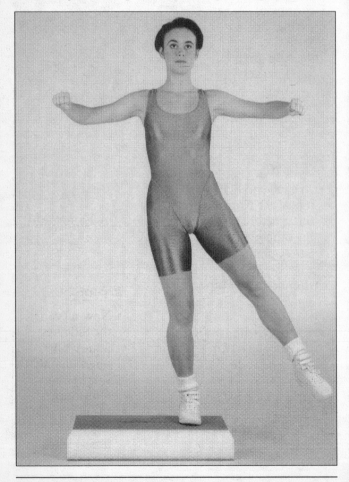

probably lean over to the opposite side, which could cause injury, or you may even over-balance.

- Repeat 16 times.

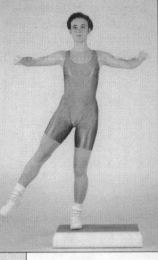

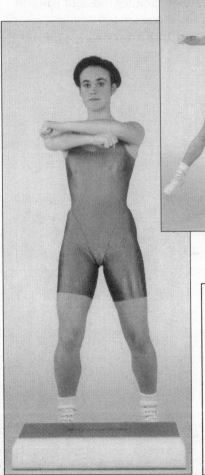

Repeaters

- Now repeat the Side Leg Squeeze 3 times on one side before returning to the other side.
- Repeat 8 times.

Leg Curl

- Substitute the Side Leg Squeeze with a Lower Leg Curl (a kick-your-bottom action).
- Safety points: Don't fling your leg. Control your leg on the curl-in and the lowering-down, to get the most out of the exercise. Think about the back of your thigh, which is the area you are working, and perform the exercise with control.
- Repeat 16 times.

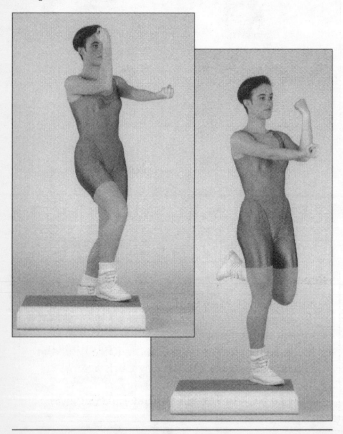

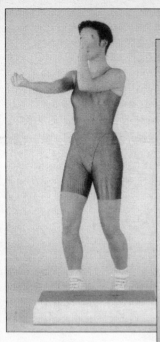

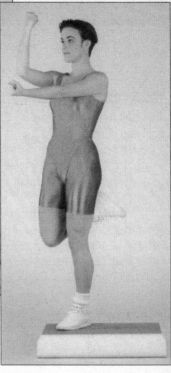

Repeaters

- Now repeat the Leg Curl 3 times at each end of the step.
- Repeat this 8 times.
- If you feel able to, go through the Knee Lifts, the Side Leg Squeezes and the Leg Curls again, including all the Repeaters.
- Now go back to Travelling Knee Lifts (singles).

Combination

At each end of the step perform:
- 1 Knee Lift;
- 1 Side Leg Squeeze;
- 1 Leg Curl.

Try the arms with this if you can:
- Knee Raise – arms go up at the point of the lift;
- Side Leg Squeeze – arms in a Shoulder Pull-Back as the leg goes out to the side;
- Leg Curl - arms in a Bicep Curl.

Repeat this combination 8 times. Don't get frustrated if you can't match the arms with the legs straightaway as the co-ordination is difficult and you may take a little while to get used to it.

Leg Flicks

- Right foot on to the step.
- Flick the left leg.
- Right foot back down on to the floor and tap.

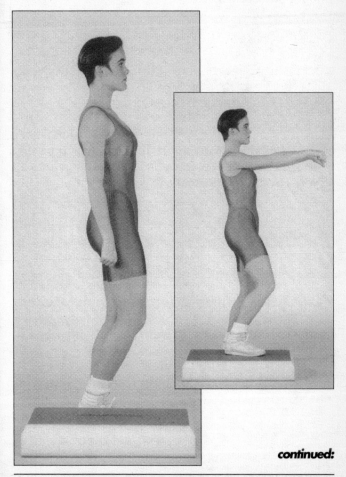

continued:

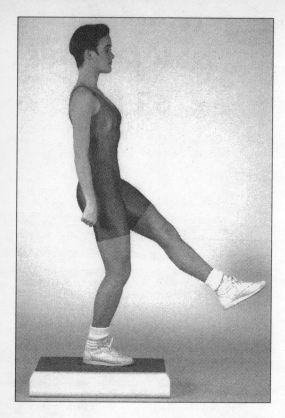

- Repeat this with the right leg leading 3 times (i.e., 3 Leg Flicks).
- Safety points: Flick the leg with control – no need to lock out the knee.
- Keep the standing leg (on the step) slightly bent.
- **Optional arms**: Front Shoulder Raise, as shown.

Over the Top

- Step over to the other side of the step.
- Right foot goes on to the step first.

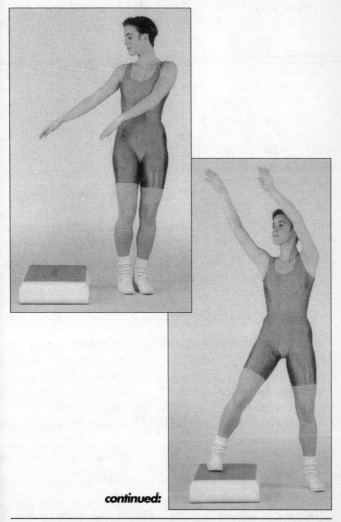

continued:

- You can put a jump into this move if you feel confident and energetic. If not, just step over.
- You are now on the other side of your step.
- **Optional arms**: Circle your arms as you travel over the step.
- Repeat the 3 Leg Flicks, only this time your left leg will lead.

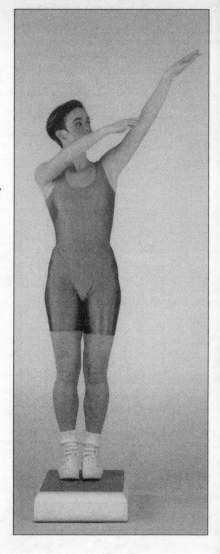

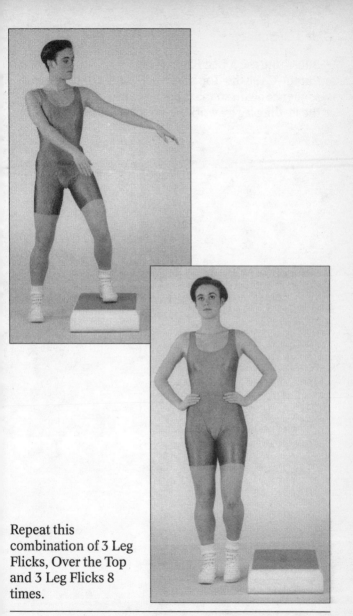

Repeat this combination of 3 Leg Flicks, Over the Top and 3 Leg Flicks 8 times.

Side Leg Squeezes

- Substitute the 3 Leg Flicks with 3 Side Leg Squeezes.
- Put the Over-the-Top movement in the middle of the sequence again so that you are continually changing the leading leg by working from both sides of the step.

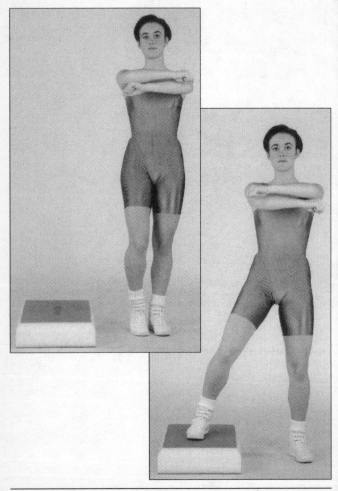

- Safety point: Keep upright rather than leaning to one side on the Side Leg Squeeze.
- Repeat 8 times.

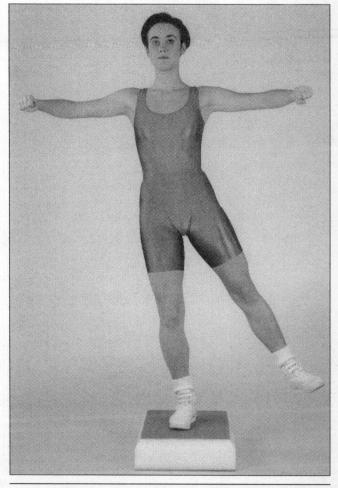

Leg Curl

- Substitute the 3 Side Leg Squeezes with 3 Leg Curls and put an Over-the-Top movement in the middle.
- Repeat 8 times.

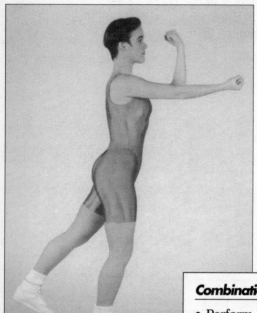

Combination

- Perform 1 Leg Flick, 1 Side Leg Squeeze and 1 Leg Curl before going Over the Top.
- Perform the same combination from the other side of the step.
- Repeat 8 times.

COOLING DOWN

Over the Top Lengthways

- Stand at the end of your step facing forwards.
- Carefully step Over the Top.
- You can add a jump to this movement if you feel
  energetic enough by this stage!

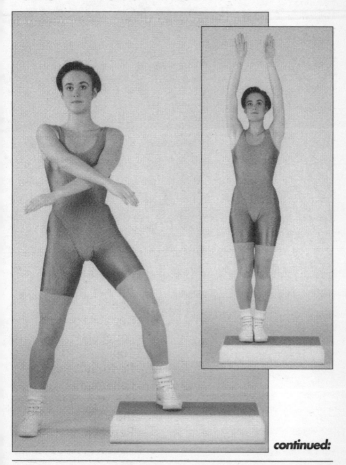

continued:

- Gradually bring this Over the Top to a very slow step across allowing your body to wind down and your breathing to become normal again.

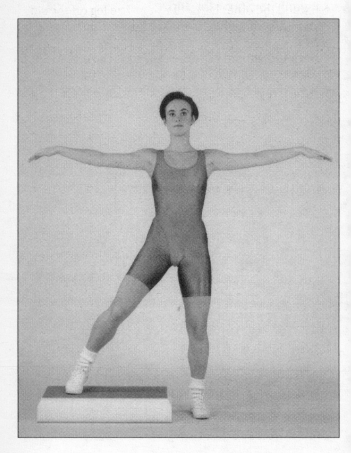

Groin Stretch

- From the Over the Top exercise leave one foot on the step.
- Your hips should be facing forwards.
- Extend the other leg to the side. The leg on the step should be straight and the leg on the floor should be bent.
- Both feet should be turned towards the corners of the room (toes should be turned outwards).
- You should feel a stretch in your inside thigh on your straight leg.
- Hold for about 8 seconds.

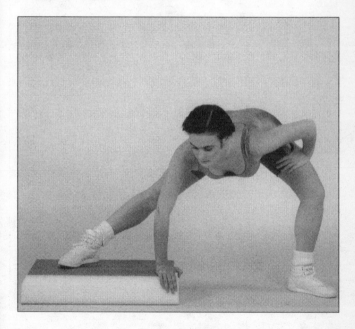

Calf Stretch

- Swivel your hips and feet around to face in from the end of the step.
- The leg on the step should be bent, and the leg extended behind should be straight.
- Your heel should be pushed down towards the floor.
- You should feel the stretch at the back of your lower leg (calf).
- Hold for about 8 seconds.

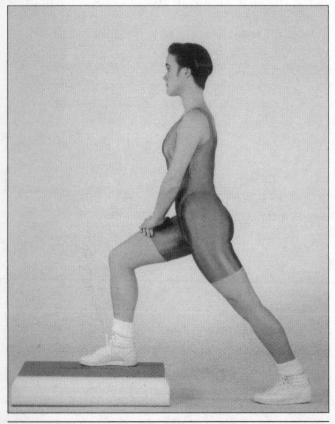

Front Thigh Stretch

- From the Calf Stretch position, drop the knee of your extended leg and push your hip on that side forward.
- If you wish you can drop your knee right down to the floor, but you may need a mat to support it.
- Hold for about 8 seconds.

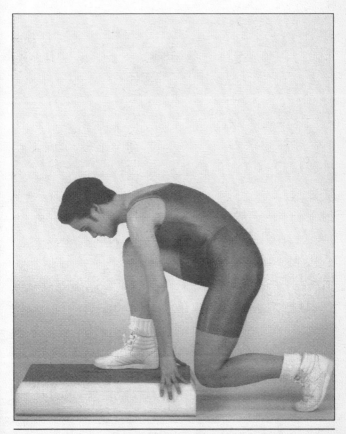

Back of Thigh (Hamstring) Stretch

- Stand up from the Hip Flexor Stretch and bend the leg on the floor.
- Straighten the leg that is on the step.
- Lean forward from your hips with a straight back, only as far as is comfortable.
- You should feel a stretch in the back of your thigh.
- Hold the stretch for about 8 seconds.

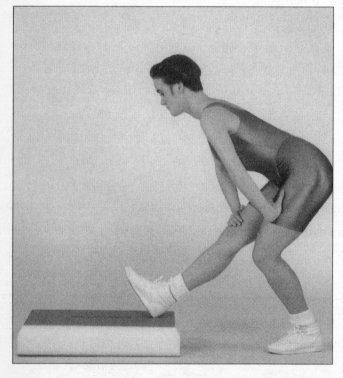

Repeat the Groin Stretch, the Calf Stretch, the Front Thigh Stretch and the Back of Thigh Stretch on the other side of your step.

Underarm (Tricep) Stretch

- Bend your elbow and place your hand behind your shoulder blades, as shown.
- Apply a gentle pressure with your other hand.
- Hold for about 8 seconds.
- Repeat on the other arm.

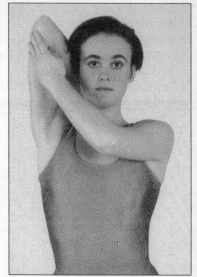

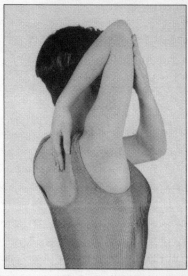

Chest Stretch

- Clasp your hands behind your back and squeeze your shoulder blades together.
- Hold for about 8 seconds.

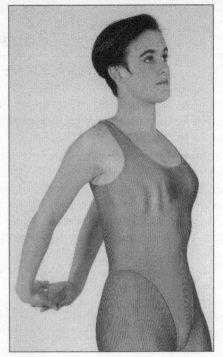

It is important to complete your step workout with the Cooling-Down Stretches, particularly if you decide to finish your workout here for today, and are not going on to the Tum and Back exercises. The stretches will ease out the muscles that have become shortened through working hard, and they will also reduce the possibility of soreness later on.

I hope you enjoyed your step challenge. For a summary of all the exercises, see pages 216 to 218.

CHAPTER 7
Advanced Dyna-Step Challenge

INCREASING THE PACE

It may be several weeks or months before you feel ready to take on the Advanced Challenge. It doesn't matter how long it takes before you can progress as you will be able to gain quite a high level workout from the New Stepper's Challenge. You can do this by increasing the number of repetitions on movements, by making your movements larger and more energetic, and perhaps by making your arm movements more energetic. You must feel comfortable with all of the steps in the New Stepper's Challenge and feel able to cope with the intensity without too many stresses and strains before you progress to the Advanced Challenge.

When you first 'attack' the routines in this Advanced Dyna-Step Challenge, keep to low repetitions of movements, maybe half of those suggested, and pace through the exercises without music before you expect yourself to perform at a faster speed. If the choreography really does feel too complicated at first, just introduce one or two of the steps into your New Stepper's Challenge and learn them gradually, without affecting your workout too much. In fact, this Advanced Challenge is an extension of the New Stepper's Challenge, so a lot of the material will be familiar to you.

Remember the health guidelines discussed on page 44. Look at these again, particularly if you are skipping the New Stepper's Challenge and coming straight in at this advanced level.

Also note that you should never feel *any* pain or discomfort when stepping and that you should *always* work within a comfortable level. When performing the Advanced Challenge for the first time, however physically fit you are, work on a low step of five or six inches until you become used to the movement patterns. It may only take one or two sessions before you feel competent enough to increase your step height.

Warm up first with the sequence in Chapter 5; however experienced you are at stepping you still need to perform a thorough warm-up. Don't forget to have a towel and some drinking water near to hand.

Ready to go?

This section is shorter in relation to the New Stepper's Challenge.

Single Heel Digs on the Step – Bicep Curl Arms

- As in the New Stepper's Challenge, but using Bicep Curl Arms.
- Safety points: Think about your posture at the start of your workout. If you stand tall now you are more likely to maintain your posture throughout the workout; i.e., start as you mean to carry on!
- Try 8 repetitions.

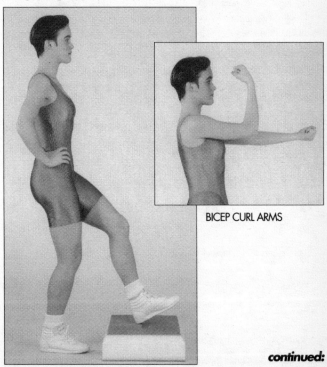

BICEP CURL ARMS

continued:

Single Toe Taps on the Step – Pec Dec Arms

- As in New Stepper's Challenge, but using Pec Dec Arms.
- Try 8 repetitions.

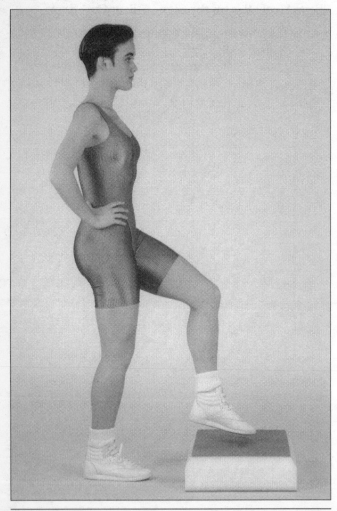

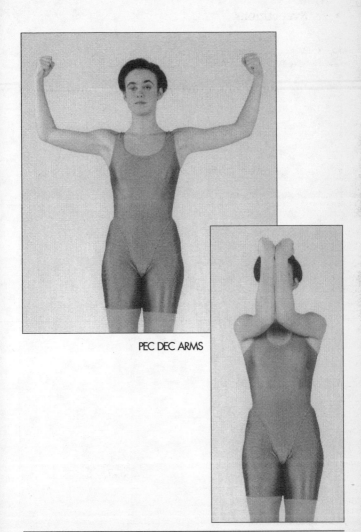

PEC DEC ARMS

March on Top of the Step and March on the Floor

- As in New Stepper's Challenge, but using Bicep Curl Arms.
- Try 8 repetitions.

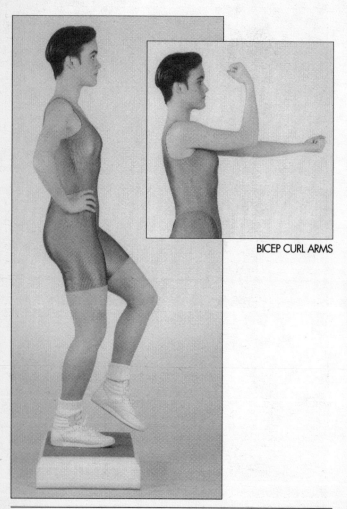

BICEP CURL ARMS

Simple Step – Right-Leg Lead

• Try 4 repetitions.

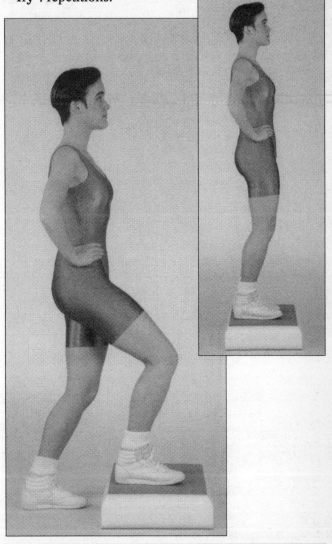

Simple Step – Left-Leg Lead

- Try 4 repetitions.
- Decrease these repetitions to 2 reps right leg and 2 reps left leg. Then,

Alternating Tap-Down Step

- As in the New Stepper's Challenge. This is the step that forms the basis for a lot of other movements. Repeat this step until you feel completely comfortable with the rhythm.
- Don't use your arms at the moment.

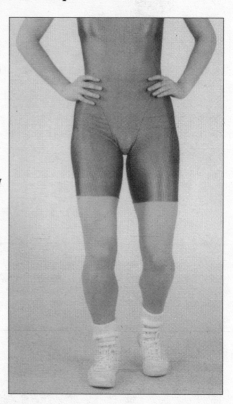

V-Step Combination

- V-Step with right-leg lead.
- **Optional arms**: Alternate Shoulder Pull-Backs (using the same arm as legs).

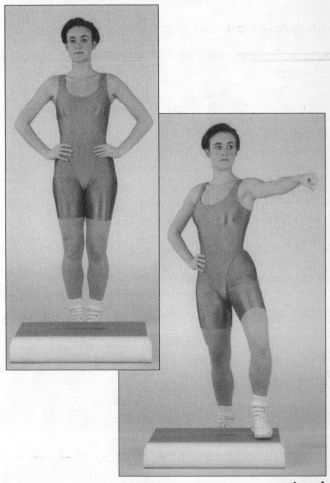

continued:

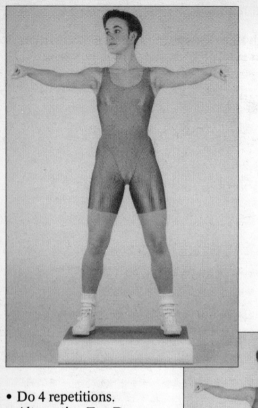

- Do 4 repetitions.
- Alternating Tap-Down Change, right-leg lead.
- **Optional arms**: Front Shoulder Raises .
- Do 4 repetitions.
- Reduce this down to 2 V-Steps and 2 Alternating Tap-Down Steps.
- Repeat a few times.

Knee Lifts

- Begin with Knee Lifts to the front but travel this movement across the step as soon as you can.

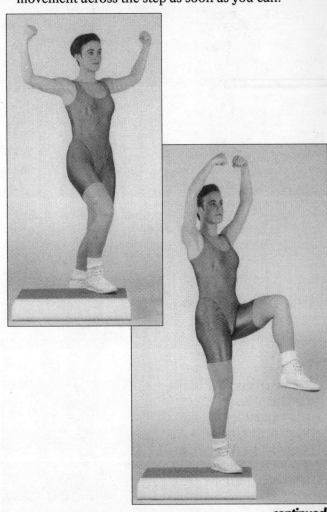

continued:

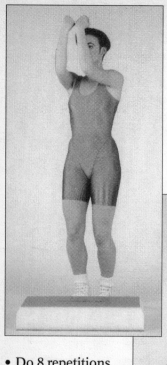

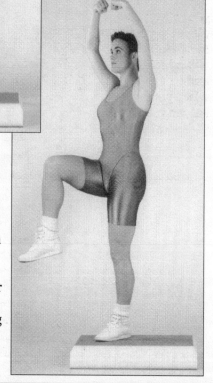

- Do 8 repetitions (4 each end of the step).
- Safety points: Your back must remain straight on the knee-lifting part of the movement. If your back arches you may be attempting to lift your leg too high.

- **Optional:** Add a jump while your foot is on the step and pushing your body weight up into the Knee Lift. If you add the jump the whole of your foot should land back on the step; i.e., don't land with your toes only. Land with your whole foot placed securely on the step. The jump will add intensity and can be used when you need to get more out of your workout.

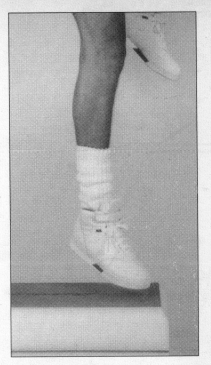

Repeaters

- Perform 3 Knee Lifts at each end of the step (maybe with jumps).
- Do 8 repetitions (4 sets of 3 lifts at each end of the step).
- The same safety points for Knee Lifts, opposite, apply.

Side Leg Squeeze

- Travel across the step performing 1 Side Leg Squeeze at each end. You may wish to jump, as in the Knee Lifts.
- Do 8 repetitions altogether.
- **Optional arms**: Arms overhead for each Knee Lift, with Pec Dec (see page 77) in between (bridging movement).
- Safety points: Keep upright as you take your leg out to the side. It may be tempting to lean in the opposite direction as you lift your leg out to the side. There is no need to lift your leg too high.

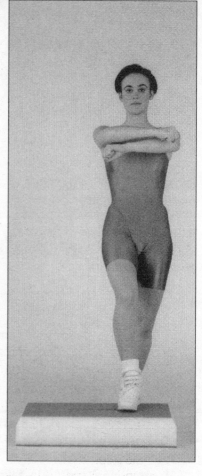

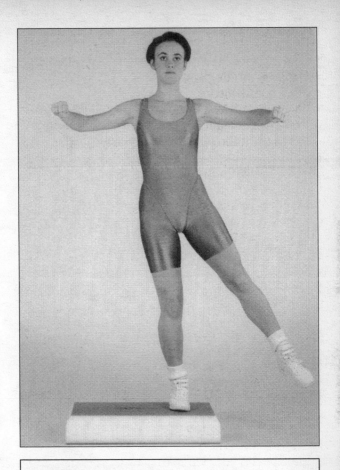

Repeaters

- Perform 3 Side Leg Squeezes at each end of the step.
- Optional arms: Shoulder Pull-Backs as your leg goes out to the side. Hands roll in between each movement.
- Do 8 repetitions.

Leg Curl

- Curl your leg behind you at each end of the step.
- **Optional arms:** Bicep Curls.
- Try 8 repetitions.
- Safety points: Control your leg as you let it down from the curl. Get maximum effect from the exercise by concentrating on the back of your thigh.

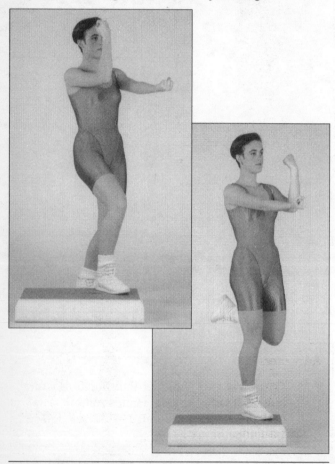

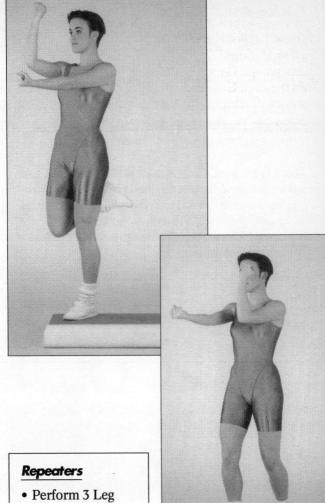

Repeaters

- Perform 3 Leg Curls at each end of the step.
- 8 repetitions.

Combination

At each end of the step perform:

- 1 Knee Lift;
- 1 Side Leg Squeeze;
- 1 Leg Curl.
- Do 8 repetitions.
- Get used to the leg pattern first and then add the arms for each of the 3 movements.

There is no need to repeat all of the above, as you did in the New Stepper's Challenge. We will now go into some more advanced movements in terms of co-ordination and intensity. So far the Advanced Dyna-Step Challenge will have taken you about 8 to 10 minutes.

Leg Flicks

- Right leg on to the step and tap on top of the step with your left leg (up tap, down tap).
- Once you have got used to this step make the tap on top of the step a low Leg Flick (up flick, down tap).
- Safety points: Keep the flick low and retain an upright posture.
- **Optional arms:** Front Shoulder Raises (see page 81).
- Perform 3 Leg Flicks.

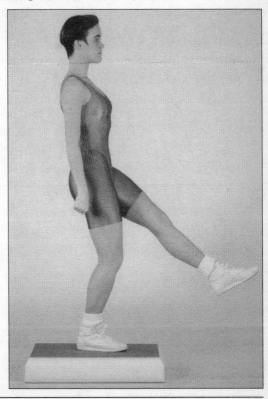

Over the Top

- Step or jump over to the other side of the step.
- **Arm movements**: Arm circles as shown, or a breaststroke action above your head.
- Perform 1 Over-the-Top step, so that you are now working from the other side of your step.
- Perform 3 Leg flicks with your left leg leading now.

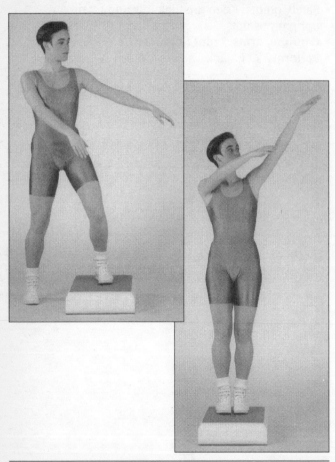

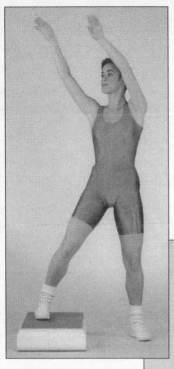

Repeat this combination of 3 Leg Flicks and an Over the Top step 4 times (2 on each side of the step).

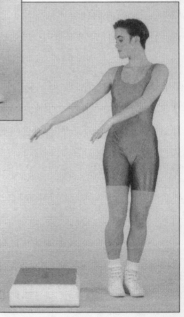

Side Leg Squeezes

- These are performed as before (see page 104) only from the side of your step (up, leg out to the side, down, tap).
- Perform 3 Side Leg Squeezes then step or jump Over the Top to repeat on the other side.

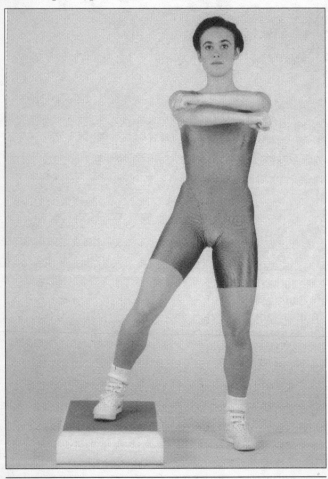

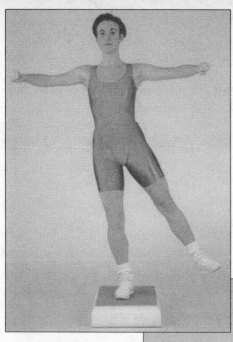

- Perform 2
  sequences on each
  side, or 4 in total.
- **Arm movements**:
  Same as the
  previous Side Leg
  Squeezes (Shoulder
  Pull-Back, with a
  Hand Roll in
  between).

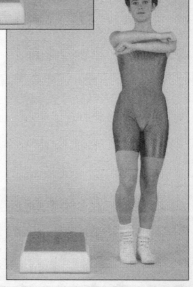

Leg Curl

- Right leg leading – 3 Leg Curls then step or jump
  Over the Top to repeat from the other side with a left
  leg lead.
- **Arm movements**: As before, Bicep Curls.
- Repeat 4 times.

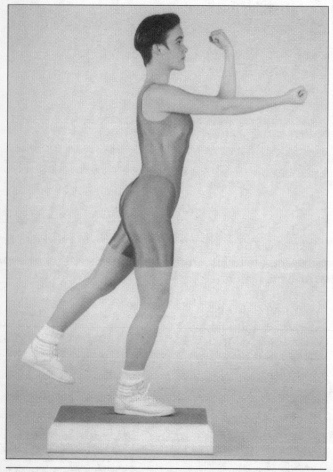

Combination

At each end of the step perform:

- 1 Leg Flick;
- 1 Side Leg Squeeze;
- 1 Leg Curl;
- 1 Over the Top.
- Repeat 8 times (4 sequences on each side of the step).

Jumps on all of these steps are optional. There is an increased risk of injury if jumps are not performed with caution. They will also elevate your heart rate and cause the workload to increase. Make sure that you feel ready for this!

Upside-Down V-Step – Right-Leg Lead

- From the end of your step, step up and place the whole of your foot securely on the far end of the step.
- Bring the other foot up to join it.
- Step back down with the leading leg, then bring the other foot down.
- You have now made an upside-down 'V'.
- Perform 4 with the right leg always leading.

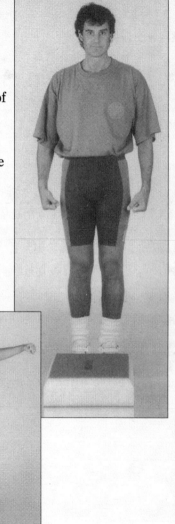

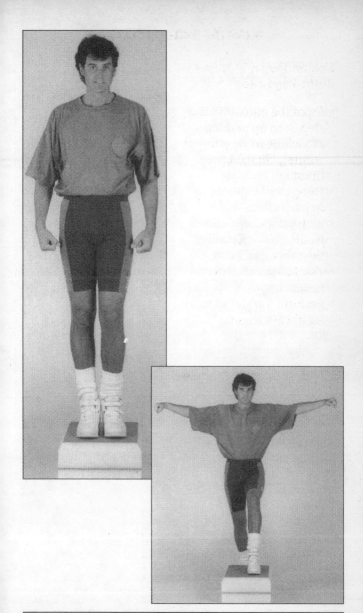

Upside-Down V-Step – Left-Leg Lead

- Do a Tap-Down Change so that the left leg now leads.
- Perform 4 repeats of the Upside-Down V-Step.
- Gradually, when you feel comfortable with the rhythm of the step, change to 2 Upside-Down V-Steps with right-leg lead and then 2 with the left leg leading.
- Now decrease to an alternating Tap-Down Upside-Down V-Step.

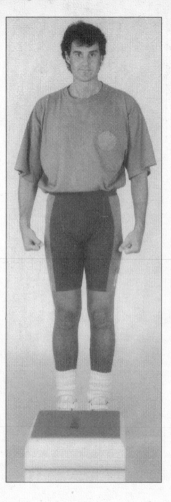

Tap-Down Change

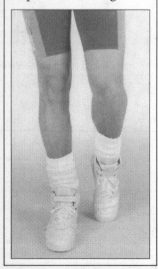

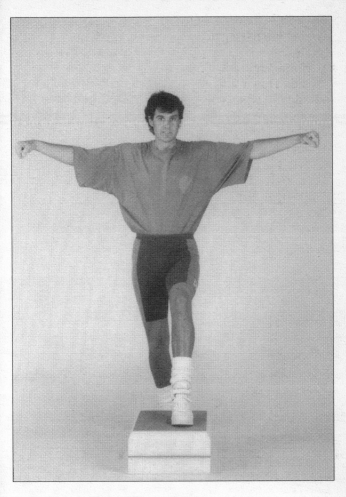

- **Optional arms:** Side Shoulder Raises.
- Perform 8 repetitions of this Alternating Lead Step.

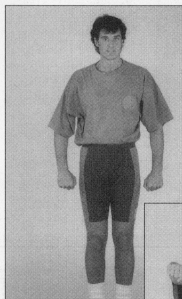

Diagonal Walk

- Walk diagonally across your step, right leg leading.
- **Optional arms**: Front Shoulder Raises.

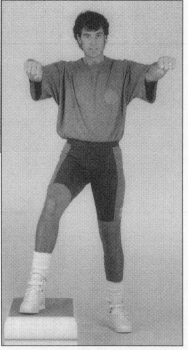

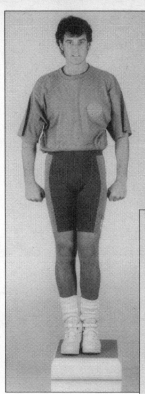

- Safety points: As you walk diagonally across, make sure that you step off at the side corner of your step. Do not step down forwards from your step as the impact of such a descent is great and potentially dangerous.
- Perform 1 Diagonal Walk.

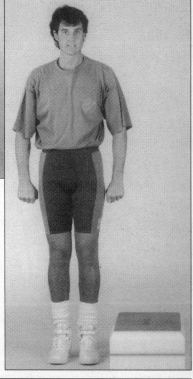

Knee Lifts Travelling Back

- Up, knee lift, down, tap.
- Perform 3 of these Knee Lifts, gradually working your way to the back of the step.

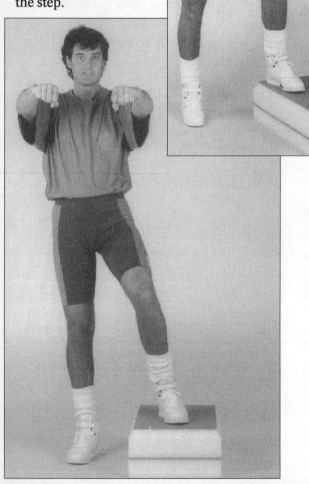

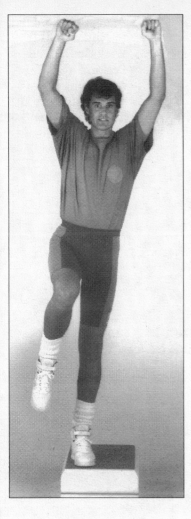

- **Arm movements**: The same as for other Knee Lifts (arms overhead on the Knee Lift, with a Pec Dec [see page 77] in between).
- You are now ready to perform another Diagonal Walk with your left leg leading so the combination will be reversed.

Repeaters

- Perform Diagonal Walk, right-leg lead.
- 3 Knee Lifts Travelling Back.
- Diagonal Walk, left-leg lead.
- 3 Knee Lifts Travelling Back.
- Repeat the whole sequence 4 times.

Diagonal Walk and Side Leg Squeezes Back

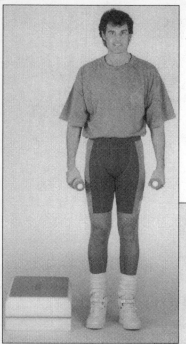

- **Arm movements**: Shoulder Pull-Backs, as before.
- Perform 4 repetitions of the whole sequence, as above (Diagonal Walk and 3 Side Leg Squeezes Travelling Back).

Steve has decided to pick up his two-pound handweights now. He is used to the step movements and is very fit. He is able to control his movements and therefore control the quality of the arm exercises and decrease any risk of injury. You will get a very good workout

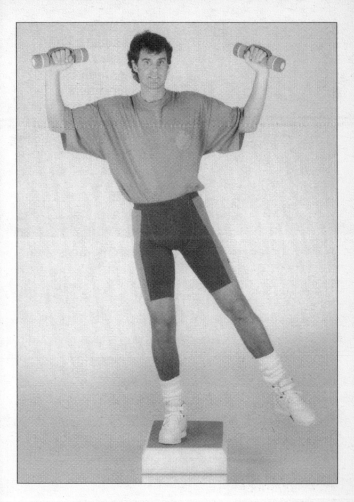

without using handweights so think carefully about
whether or not they are suitable for you.

continued:

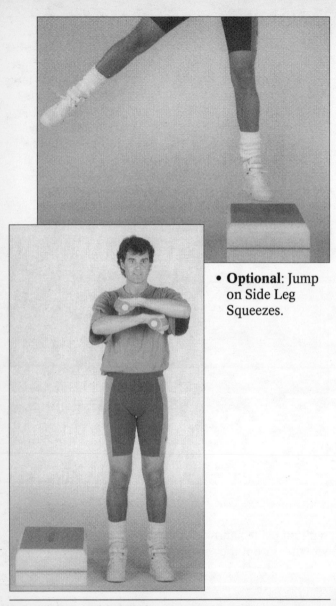

- **Optional**: Jump on Side Leg Squeezes.

Diagonal Walk and Leg Curls Travelling Back

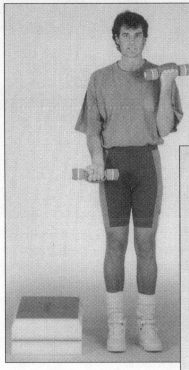

Again Steve is able to use weights, as this is a short-lever (bent arm), safe and comfortable arm movement.

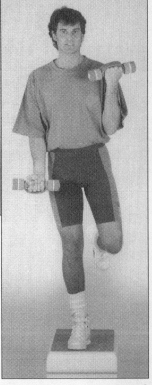

continued:

- **Optional:** Jump on the Leg Curl.
- Perform the sequence (Diagonal Walk and 3 Leg Curls back) 4 times.

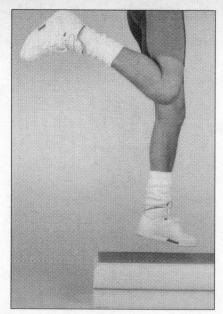

Combination

All travelling backwards on the step, perform:

- Diagonal Walk;
- 1 Knee Lift;
- 1 Side Leg Squeeze;
- 1 Leg Curl.
- Repeat 4 times.

Repeat from the Leg Flicks (page 143) once through again.

T-Step

- Step up from the end of your step with your right leg leading.

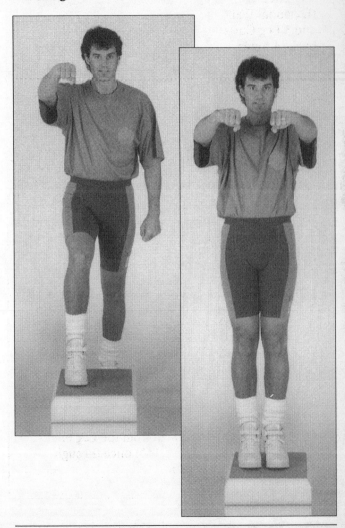

• Straddle down with your right leg first.

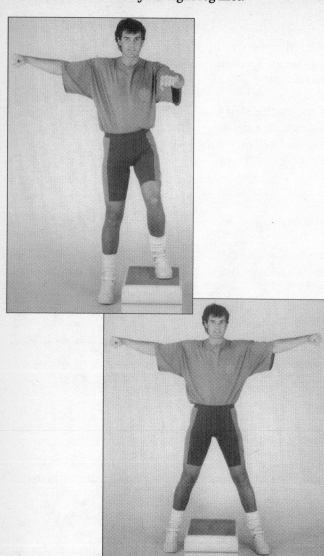

- Straddle up, right foot first (or optional jump).
- Return to the end of your step. You will have made a T-shape.
- Perform this step 4 times with a right-leg lead and then 4 times with a left-leg lead.
- Remember that the jump is optional.
- Gradually drop down to 2 complete T-Steps, with a right lead, and 2 with a left lead.
- Now alternate the right and left lead to make an alternating T-Step.
- Perform 8 T-Steps.

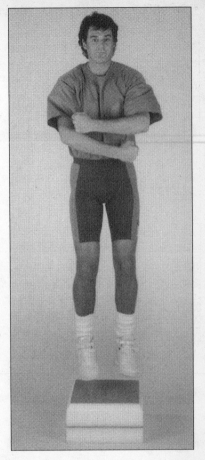

- **Optional arms**: On the step up from the end of the step do a single front Shoulder Raise (same arm as leg).

This is where the pace really increases!

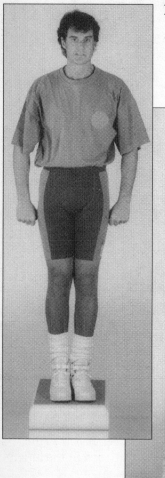

Power Lunges

- Right leg out to the side in a lunge.

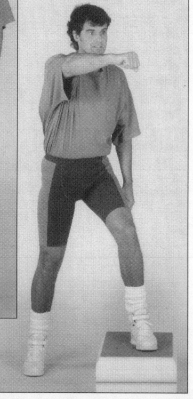

- Left leg out to the side in a lunge.
- Perform 8 Lunges.
- Safety points: Lunges can be very strenuous. It is important that your technique is correct. Only place your toe lightly on the floor as it touches for the lunge. The leg that remains on the step should remain slightly bent.

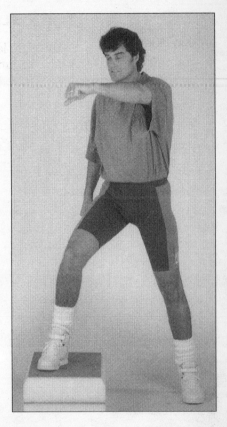

- **Arm movements**: This is quite an easy one because it feels completely natural. Arm punches across the body (opposite arm to the leg extended in the lunge).

Power Squats

- From the top of your step, squat to the right and hold for 3 counts. On the fourth bring your leg back on to the step.
- From the top.
- Right squat.

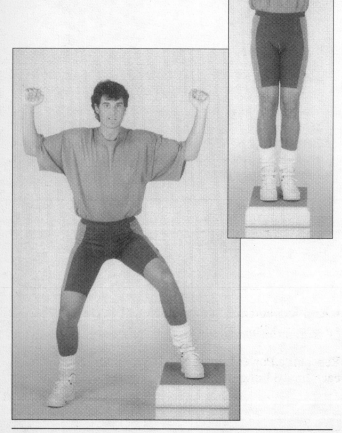

• Left squat.

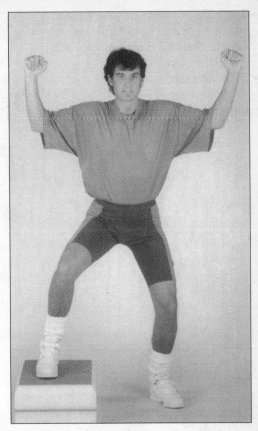

- **Arm movements**: Slow and strong Pec Dec.
- Perform 4 Power Squats.

Repeat the Power Lunges and Squats another 3 times – each time 8 Lunges and 4 Power Squats.

Turn Step

- This turn step is a half-turn so that you remain on the same side of the step.
- Left foot up.
- Right foot up, making almost a V-Step.

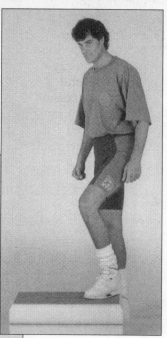

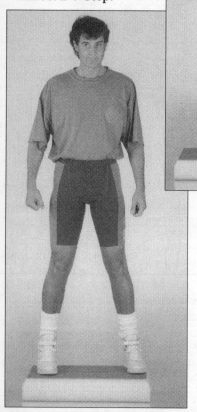

- Right foot down.
- Left foot down to finish.
- Perform 4 turns.
- Safety points: Some people get dizzy turning several times in succession. Practise this turn a lot before you attempt to perform it at speed.

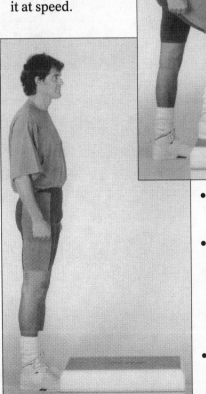

- Now change the lead leg to the right.
- **Arm movements:** Same as for V-Step, punch singly in side Shoulder Raise (same arm as leg, see page 134).
- Perform 4 turns.

Over the Top

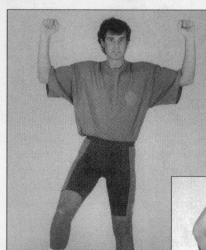

- Right foot up.
- Left foot joins on top of the step.

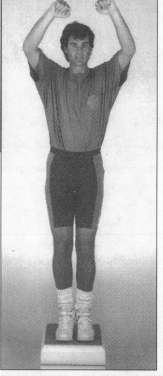

- Right foot down on the other side of the step.
- Left foot joins to finish.
- Perform 4 Over-the-Top steps, with or without a jump.
- **Arm movements**: Breaststroke arms overhead.

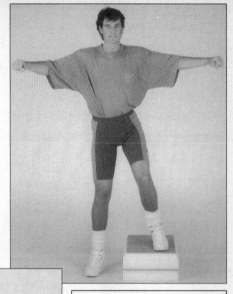

Repeaters

- Now reduce the Turn Step to 2 turns.
- Reduce the Over the Top to 2.
- The challenge will be whether or not you are able to perform one of each.
- 1 Half-Turn.
- 1 Over the Top, ending up on the other side of the step.
- Perform 8 times, alternating the steps.

Combination

- Diagonal Walk.
- Turn Step: a small one so that you end up in the middle of your step rather than at the end.
- Over the Top.
- Lunges or more strenuous Jumping Jacks.

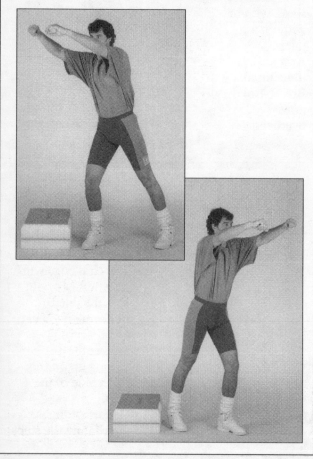

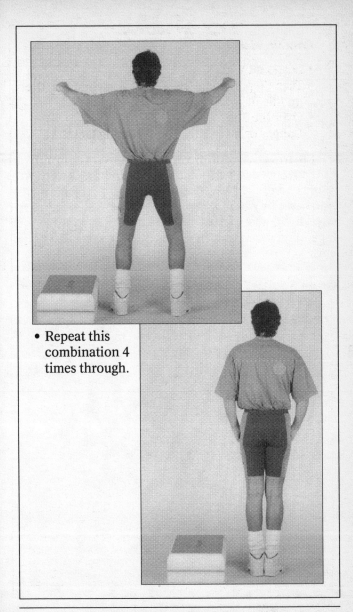

- Repeat this combination 4 times through.

COOLING DOWN

Repeat the sequence at the beginning of the workout
(see page 127–30, Step Familiarization).
- Heel Digs and Toe Taps, 8 repetitions of each.
- Marches on the top of the step and on the floor.
- Gradually slowing down so that your heart rate
  returns to pre-exercise level.

You now need to perform the same stretches as shown
at the end of the New Stepper's Challenge. Don't try to
skip these or you'll probably be unable to step for a few
days; tight, unstretched muscles are more prone to
injury and soreness. These stretches are essential. They
are:

Groin Stretch

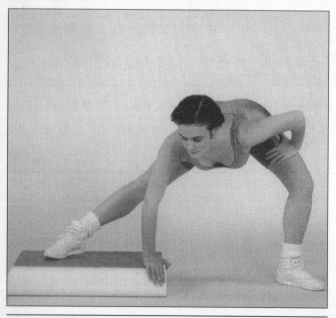

**Calf
Stretch**

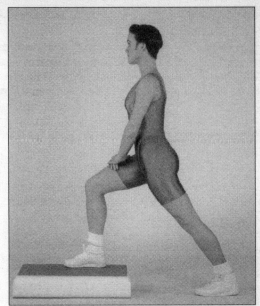

**Front
Thigh
Stretch**

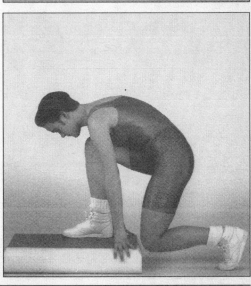

Back of Thigh Stretch

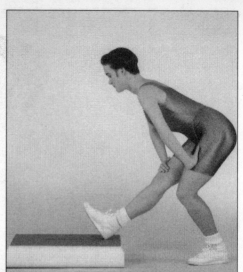

Underarm Stretch

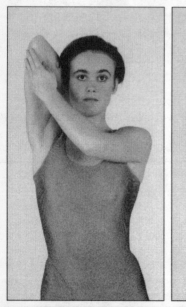
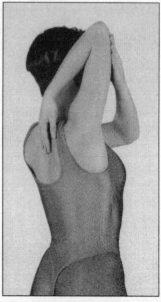

Chest Stretch

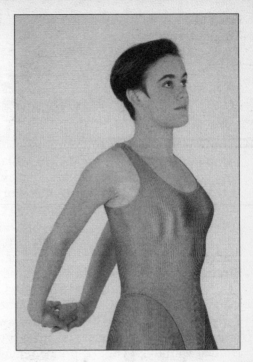

You may have completed your exercise for the day, or you may wish to continue with the Tum and Back exercises.

CHAPTER 8
Tight Tums and Healthy Backs

Stepping is more or less a complete workout for most of your body's major muscle groups. After only a few weeks you will notice the tightening effect on your bottom, thighs and lower-leg muscles. You won't develop huge muscles and be able to enter body-building contests, but your muscles will have a tighter, more defined appearance and hopefully give smaller readings on your tape measure.

Your upper-back and arm muscles will also improve in tone and appearance if you are able to perform the arm exercises in a controlled way. At first you will be concentrating on the leg movements, but when you become familiar with those your co-ordination might stretch to managing the arm movements at the same time! You will not necessarily have to add the handweights to work your arms and upper body successfully.

The areas that may be neglected when stepping are your abdominal and back muscles. Everyone is aware of the necessity for abdominal exercises – most exercise programmes seem to 'blitz' this area of the body. Flat stomachs and tight waistlines are one of the most sought-after effects of exercise, and consequently, abdominal exercise positions are often well known. However, exercises for the spine (back) are often sadly neglected, and that's a great shame.

We need strong abdominal and back muscles to attain and control correct posture and body alignment.

Most back problems are a result of postural deficiencies due to weak supporting muscles. If your abdominal and spinal muscles are well exercised, strong and supportive, your spine is much more likely to be in a well-aligned position and you will experience less back pain as a result. Your stomach will look flatter simply because you are able to stand correctly!

These exercises are an essential supplement to your step challenge and if you follow them you will not only see a cosmetic improvement but will be protecting your 'Health Related Fitness' by supporting your spine in a positive way.

The exercises in this chapter are unique in that they offer the optional resistance of a Dyna-Band. If you feel able to use the Dyna-Band where suggested you will find that the exercises produce quick results, but they will not be gruelling or exhausting. Try the exercises without a Dyna-Band first and then gradually introduce the added resistance as you feel the need for more challenging exercises.

These exercises can be performed after your step challenge or, if you have decided to split up the workout into two shorter sections, you could perform these exercises after a warm-up and leave your step challenge for the alternate days.

We are using the Dyna-Step in this section. Another type of step may not be as comfortable to lie on, so to protect your spine, and to make the exercises more comfortable you could either purchase a step mat or place a thin mat or towel over your step. If these suggestions don't work, lie on the floor on a mat or towel (you will be unable to use the Dyna-Band for some of the positions when on the floor).

The Dyna-Step is made up of two pieces that slot together rather like Lego bricks. We have separated the two parts and placed them in a T-shape, with the smaller half forming the top of the T. Steve fits quite comfortably on the T-shape, and he is over six feet tall. Nicky has no problems at all and found the positions extremely comfortable.

Select the level of exercises that you feel happy with. You should experience no pain or discomfort. Do not force yourself to complete the suggested repetitions if you feel tired. The idea is that you progressively build up to the more difficult exercises with the Dyna-Band and eventually reach the suggested number of repetitions.

Abdominal Curl – Without Dyna-Band

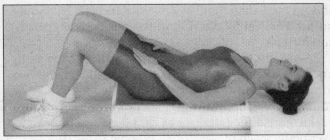

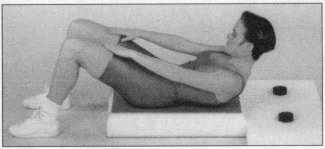

- Lie on your step with your knees bent and your feet flat on the floor. Make sure that your bottom is fully on the step and not just wedged on the edge.
- Either slide your hands up your thighs, or place them behind your head (the second option is slightly harder).
- Gently raise your head and shoulders off the step using your abdominal muscles to lift you.
- Lower down with control.
- Perform 16 repetitions.
- Safety points: Push your lower back into the step.
- Breathe out as you lift up.
- Try not to pull up with your neck. If your abdominal muscles are not strong, only attempt to lift your shoulders just off the step – even this small lift will be effective.

Abdominal Curl – With Dyna-Band

- Place the Dyna-Band – keeping it as wide as possible so that it doesn't twist up when you exercise – under your step as shown.
- Your body weight will fix it in place.
- Bend your knees and place your feet flat on the floor.
- Take the ends of the Dyna-Band, one in each hand, and pull them over your shoulders.

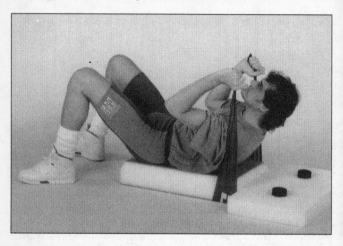

- Pulling the Dyna-Band up with you, gradually curl up as before, just lifting your head and shoulders off the floor.
- Perform 12 repetitions.
- Safety points: As before.

Pec Dec – Without Dyna-Band

- Lie on your back on the step
- With control bring your bent arms into the middle of your chest and lower them back down.
- This exercise will work your chest (pectoral) muscles, the muscles that support women's breasts.
- Perform 16 repetitions.

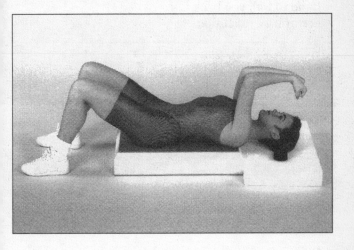

Pec Dec – With Dyna-Band

- Thread the Dyna-Band under your step, keeping it as flat as possible.
- Take one end in each hand under your armpits.
- Slowly bring in your elbows to the middle of your chest.
- Safety point: As you lower yourself back down, control the movement and don't allow the Dyna-Band to pull you back.
- Perform 12 repetitions.

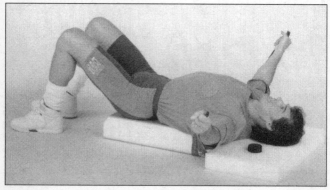

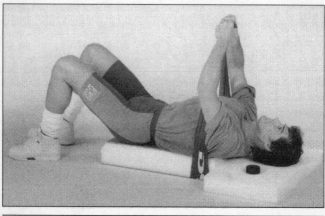

Waist Twist – Without Dyna-Band

- In the same position as for the Abdominal Curl, lying on your back with your knees bent and feet flat on the floor.
- Bring one hand across to the opposite knee and then lower down with control.
- Now repeat on the other side.
- Repeat 16 times (8 on each side).
- Safety points: Breathe out as you lift across. Keep the small of your back pressed into the floor.
- Reach across and not up so that you feel your waist muscles working.

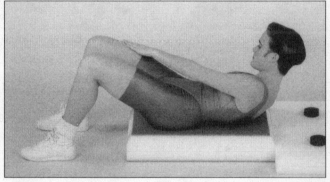

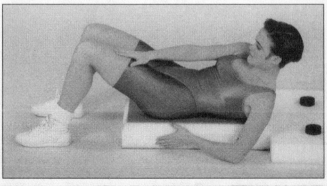

Waist Twist – With Dyna-Band

- Place your Dyna-Band under your step as shown.
- Hold both ends of the band in either hand and reach with one hand across to the opposite knee as above.
- The Dyna-Band requires more force or effort and your waist muscles will have to work harder.
- Repeat 12 times (6 on each side).

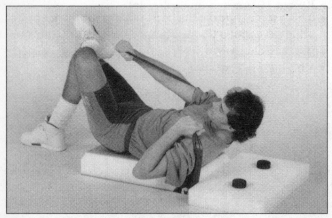

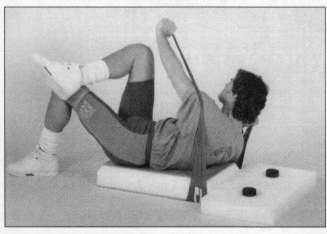

Elbow Push-Up – Beginner Level

- Sit at the end of your step with your feet flat on the floor.
- Place your arms behind you with your fingers facing towards your bottom.
- Lean back as you bend your elbows and then push back up, again taking care not to snap your elbow joint.
- This exercise works the back of your arm (tricep) which is an area that is often neglected and tends to become flabby with age.
- Perform 12 repetitions.

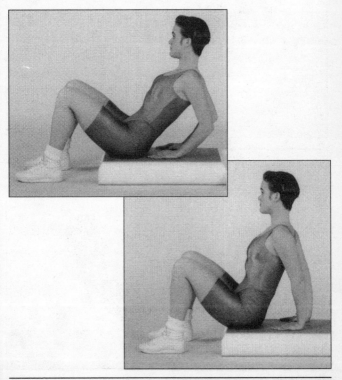

Elbow Push-Up – Intermediate

- Sitting at the end of your step as before, this time lift your bottom off the step and bend your elbows, lowering your body weight to just off the floor.
- Push up carefully, taking care not to jar your elbows.
- Repeat 8 times.
- Safety points: Fingers must face your bottom or you may damage your wrists or elbows. Bend at the elbows and not in the middle of your body.
- Stop if you feel uncomfortable; this is a strenuous exercise and your arms will be weak compared to your legs. It is, however, very effective!

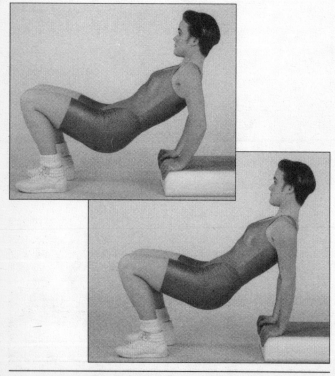

Elbow Push-Up – Advanced

- Take the same position as above, but lift one leg off the floor as well as your bottom.
- This is very demanding and really needs building up to.
- Men tend to have more strength in their upper bodies than women do and may therefore manage this exercise more easily than some women.

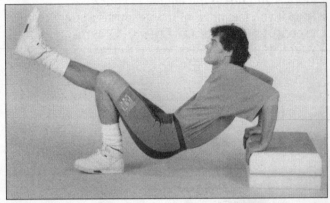

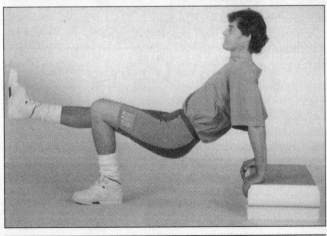

Shoulder Squeeze – Without Dyna-Band

- Lie on your tummy on your step. Your chest should be at one end of the step. You may wish to cross your ankles to keep your feet firmly fixed to the floor.
- Your body should remain still but just lift your arms behind you, squeezing your shoulder blades together.
- Release with control.
- This exercise works the upper back and is excellent if you have round shoulders that you are trying to correct.
- Repeat 8 times.

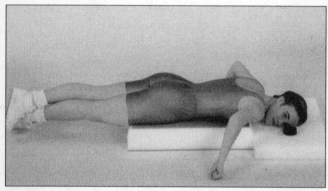

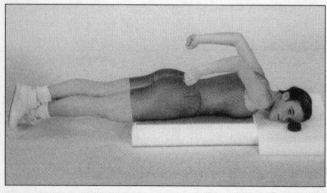

Shoulder Squeeze – With Dyna-Band

- The Dyna-Band should be lying under your step. Take the ends in either hand.
- Extend your arms behind you and squeeze your shoulder blades together.
- Repeat 8 times.
- Safety points: When using the Dyna-Band keep your elbows relaxed and perform the movement with care and control.

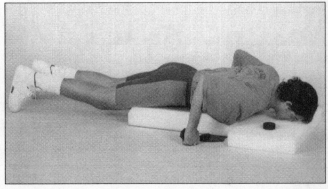

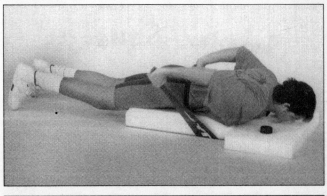

Lumbar Lift – Beginner

- Lying on your tummy as before, place your hands on your bottom.
- Raise your head and shoulders off the floor – it doesn't matter if it's only a few inches.
- Lift from your lower-back muscles.
- Repeat 6 times.
- Safety points: Do not perform this exercise if you have back problems or the exercise causes you pain in your back.
- Keep your eyes looking down at the floor the whole time so you don't over-arch your neck, which is extremely vulnerable.

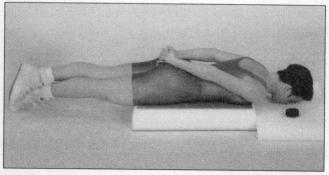

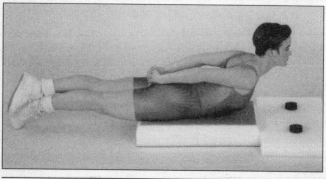

Lumbar Lift – Advanced

- In the same position as for the previous exercise, place your hands at the side of your head.
- Lift your head and shoulders off the step – it need not be very high. Keep looking at the floor throughout. This is very important.
- Lower down with control.
- Repeat 6 times.

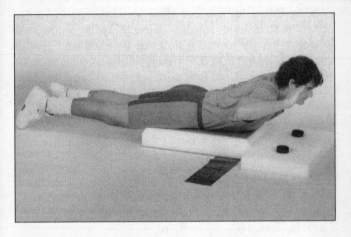

Repeat the seven exercises once or twice more, depending on your previous exercise experience. Cool-down stretches must be performed now, and you'll find these in the next chapter.

CHAPTER 9
Cooling Down

I always think that this is the best part of any workout! Cooling down allows you time to relax and to forget about the stresses and strains of everyday life. If you lead a hectic life, try to make time for yourself and slowly unwind, relaxing into the stretch positions. This section need only take about five minutes, unless you feel like performing the stretches twice through. This is very little time spent, when you consider the benefits of stretching at the end of a workout.

Those benefits include:

An increase in your flexibility.
- If your muscles are pliable you are less prone to injury. You are less likely to strain a muscle while making a sudden movement, for your muscles are more flexible, and have more 'give' in them.
- Your posture is more likely to be well balanced. This is important because postural imbalances can lead to upper- and lower-back pain.
- You should be able to complete everyday tasks with ease; for example, bending down to pick up objects, or children, or reaching up to a high shelf. Flexible people take household chores for granted but the less flexible can find them a nightmare.

Releasing muscles that have become tight through the constant activity involved in your workout.
- Often short tight muscles have a 'bulky' appearance, which most of us would prefer to avoid.

Stretching relaxes you both mentally and physically and will make you feel good about yourself and your workout.

- You will be finishing your exercise programme in a gentle and relaxed manner rather than feeling hot, sweaty and exhausted.

How far you will be able to stretch depends on your individual flexibility, which varies tremendously. You will notice that Nicky, the model in the pictures, is very flexible – but there is no need to force yourself to stretch as far as she can. Go only as far as is comfortable and stop immediately if you feel any pain in your joints.

Flexibility has a hereditary element. If your parents have naturally flexible joints then they may pass on this asset to you. This advantage is related to the shape and size of your joints and the structures that support them. Flexibility is also governed, to a certain extent, by body type and size. Those people with long, willowy limbs tend not to be super flexible because their muscles and tendons have to stretch further over longer bones. Your lifestyle can also affect your flexibility. If you sit all day at a desk, for example, and don't get much chance to walk around, your leg muscles will become shortened and inflexible.

If you have just finished the Tum and Back exercises you will have finished the section by lying on your front on the step. These Cool-Down stretches follow on nicely from this position so you will not even have to move! If you have just completed your step challenge and have finished exercising for the day, you can still perform these Cool-Down stretches if you wish to improve your flexibility. Lay on your step on your tummy, ready to relax. All of the stretches have been placed in the following order so that they flow nicely and involve as little moving around as possible.

Front Thigh (Quadricep) Stretch

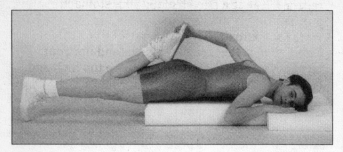

- Lying on your stomach, take your right foot in your right hand. Pull your leg gently into your bottom. Push your right hip bone into the step to increase the feel of the stretch, which should be along the front of your right thigh.
- Hold for approximately 8 seconds.
- Repeat the stretch on the left side.
- Safety points: Hold the middle part of your foot and not the end of your toes. If your knee hurts at all during this exercise, release your leg.

Abdominal Stretch

- Remain in the same position on your front.

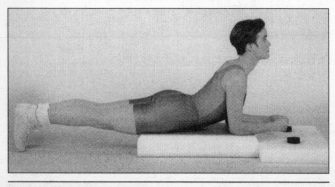

- Place your elbows on the step or floor and gently raise up, feeling a stretch along your stomach muscles.
- Hold for approximately 8 seconds.
- Safety points: Rest on your elbows and not your hands or you may attempt to push up too high and damage your lower back.
- Keep your eyes down to the floor to protect your neck.

Spinal Stretch

- This is a lovely, relaxing stretch.
- From lying on your front, push your bottom back on to your heels and stretch your arms out in front of you on the step.

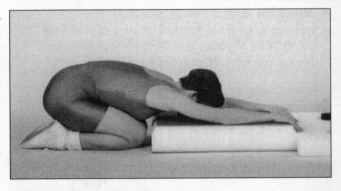

- Hold for approximately 10 seconds.
- Safety points: Keep your bottom just off of your heels to avoid excessively flexing your knees.

Back of Thigh (Hamstring) Stretch

- This is an area that tends to be very inflexible and most of us need to make an effort to stretch our hamstrings every day.
- Roll carefully on to your back and make yourself as comfortable as possible.

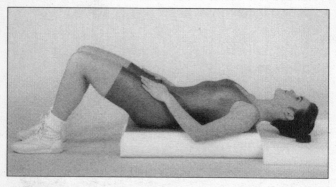

- Make sure that your bottom is fully on the step and that your neck and shoulders are relaxed.
- Bring your right knee into your chest and hold it for a few seconds.

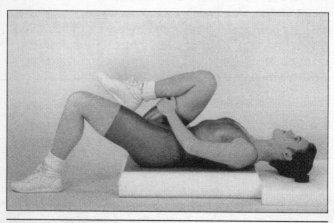

- Now extend your right leg, attempting to keep your thigh close to your chest. It is not necessary to extend your leg into a straight position - very few people are that flexible! Just extend as far as you can go comfortably. If, after a few seconds, your leg feels relaxed enough try to stretch it just a little further.

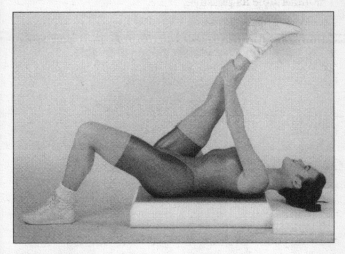

- Repeat this stretch on your right leg.
- Hold for approximately 15 to 20 seconds.
- Safety points: If the stretched leg begins to feel shaky, then lower it slightly to a less adventurous position. Your body is just telling you that you are stretching too far too quickly.

The following stretches do not necessarily have to be done if you have already performed the same stretches at the end of the step challenge.

Underarm Stretch (Tricep)

- Sit up on your step in a comfortable position. Place your arm over your head, with your hand reaching down between your shoulder blades. Apply a gentle pressure with your other arm as shown.
- Repeat on the other arm.
- Hold for approximately 8 seconds.
- Safety points: Apply pressure to your underarm and not to your elbow, which can be vulnerable.

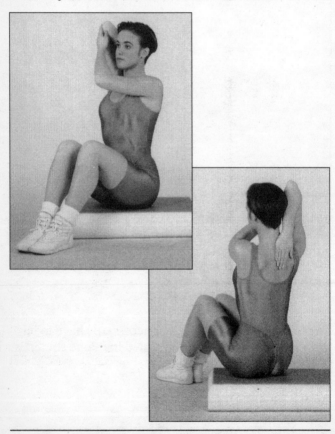

Waist Stretch

- Remain sitting on your step and reaching your arm overhead, leaning to one side.
- Place your other hand on the step for support.
- Repeat on the other side.
- Hold for approximately 8 seconds.
- Safety points: Lean directly to the side and try not to twist your body.

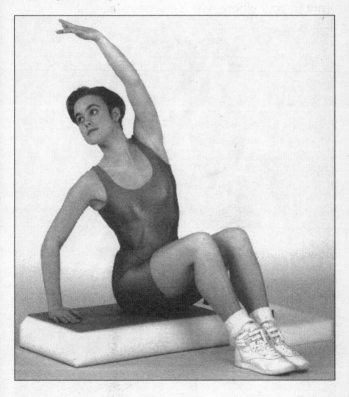

Chest Stretch

- Again, sit on your step or stand if you feel more comfortable.
- Link your hands behind your back and squeeze your shoulder blades together. You should feel a stretch across your chest.
- Hold for approximately 8 seconds.

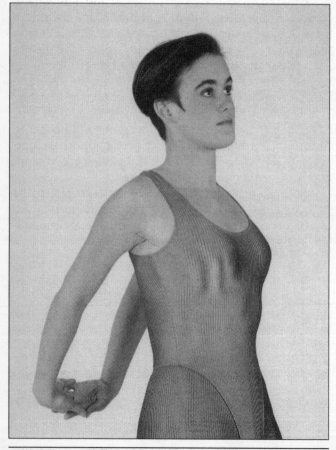

Well, that's your programme completed for today! I hope that you feel revitalized and relaxed. If you have completed your workout early in the day, you'll find you have an extra boost of energy to get you through the day's tasks. If, on the other hand, you have worked out in the evening you will have eased the tension and fatigue that a packed day can induce and you will probably sleep well.

If you begin to lose motivation and find it difficult to complete your step workout regularly try inviting a friend along to exercise with you. If you make a date to get together and work out you have more incentive to keep to that appointment when someone else is relying on you. It can also be great fun to work out the step combinations and finally to conquer the challenge together. This is why support groups, such as Weight Watchers, have such tremendous success encouraging people to stick to their programmes. We all need support, encouragement and praise at times and this idea could work well for you and your step challenge.

You may, of course, have no problems keeping to the step challenge – when you begin to see the results and experience the benefits, you will be absolutely committed. You'll probably never look back!

CHAPTER 10
Special Steppers

If you are in one of the following specialist categories check for advice and guidance in this chapter before you throw yourself into the step challenge!

STEPPING IN PREGNANCY

Exercise in pregnancy has become increasingly popular – which is great, because the benefits can be tremendous. However, caution is obviously necessary and one of the first rules to observe is this: *Pregnancy is not a time for beginning a new physical activity*.

I would strongly advise against any pregnant woman taking up stepping as a new form of exercise. For the safety of your softened and relaxed joints you need to be able to perform the step exercises competently. Any jerky or unfinished movements may jar vulnerable joints which have become loosened by hormonal changes.

Those of you who have been stepping for a while now may remember with horror how unco-ordinated you felt in those early step sessions! When your technique is poor you are much more likely to make sudden or snatched movements in order to keep up with the routine.

As a new exerciser and a pregnant mum, you would be advised to take up a non-impact form of exercise, such as swimming, and maybe enrol on a local ante- or post-natal class.

If you are pregnant, have been stepping for a while and wish to continue with your step exercise programme it will be useful for you to understand some of the physiological changes that are taking place in your body.

- An increase of approximately thirty per cent in blood volume by the twenty-fourth week of pregnancy means that your resting heart rate will be higher. When exercising, therefore, your heart is likely to beat faster for the same work level than it did in your pre-pregnant state. You may also feel more breathless when exercising. You will probably lower your effort levels gradually, and without even realizing it, as your pregnancy advances. Exercisers tend to be very good at 'listening to their bodies' and this applies even more so in pregnancy.
- Hormonal changes make the soft tissues of your joints more pliable and consequently less stable. When exercising we have to consider the weight-bearing joints, particularly in their weakened state. In stepping, the spine, hips, knees and ankles need to be considered and protected by a well-balanced programme of exercises.
- In pregnancy your centre of gravity tends to change to accommodate the bump! This can make complex movements with sudden changes in direction potentially dangerous. There is a possibility that you might lose your balance on the step!

This all sounds pretty serious but, although the physiological changes in pregnancy are remarkable, if you are sensible and moderate your exercise to feel manageable and comfortable you can safely step through your pregnancy until you no longer feel inclined to exercise – which may be at about six or seven months. If you have spent a lot of time and effort increasing your fitness levels by stepping before you became pregnant, why lose all of those benefits now? In addition to all of the regular benefits already mentioned, stepping can help you through your pregnancy by:

- Increasing the strength of your muscles to support those joints which are temporarily weakened.
- Improving your posture, enabling you to carry your baby correctly.
- Providing a low-impact exercise programme which is much easier on your joints than high-impact aerobics.
- Giving you increased energy levels (pregnancy can be very tiring).
- Increasing your self-confidence.
- Making your pregnancy happier and healthier – exercise gives you a sense of purpose, and releases endorphins which create a feeling of well-being.

If you decide that, given the benefits, you would like to continue with your step challenge during some part of your pregnancy you need to observe the following guidelines:

- Always consult with your doctor first, in the event that there are any reasons why you should not exercise in your pregnancy. This is of major importance. He or she may know of reasons why it would be unwise for you to continue to exercise; for example, hereditary factors, or high blood pressure.
- Regular step sessions of three times a week, as recommended in this programme, will be preferable to irregular stepping. Stopping and starting will only make you more prone to injury as your body will become unused to exercise during the time lapses between workouts. This is important to bear in mind, as pregnancy seems to bring erratic energy level

changes and there may be days where you do not wish to exercise. When this happens, do some very low-level activity until you feel energetic again.

Studies show that the pregnant mother can work safely at moderate levels of intensity. Maximum-intensity exercise could affect blood flow to the developing foetus. (Studies in animals have shown that high temperature increases can be passed on to the foetus, with potentially serious side-effects.) Keep exercise at a comfortable level.

- Avoid stepping in hot or humid weather.
- Start the class well hydrated by drinking a full glass of water beforehand. Drink water during the stepping phase itself and then a small fruit juice at the end of your exercise to replace lost potassium.
- Avoid bouncing, jarring or jerky exercises.
- Stick to the New Stepper's Challenge, as the Advanced Dyna-Step Challenge contains several turns, hip-shifting movements and more complicated combinations. These movements could cause misalignment to your joints.
- Use the Perceived Exertion Chart illustrated in Chapter 3 to judge how hard you are working. This will probably be more useful than monitoring your heart rate, which can be inaccurate. Remember that you should not be working at the levels that are described as being hard (i.e., 15 and above). All exercises should feel comfortable. You will have to put aside that 'Go for it' attitude you had before your pregnancy!
- As your pregnancy advances and you become heavier, more tired and less mobile, decrease your step height gradually – maybe to as little as four or five inches, depending on your fitness levels before your pregnancy.
- Stop all stepping and any other form of exercise if anything unusual occurs; for example, abdominal

cramps, joint pain or bleeding, and *see your doctor immediately*.

I regularly see pregnant women continue to step into their sixth and seventh months of pregnancy with no ill-effects, only positive benefits. These same women have also very quickly regained their fitness levels – and their figures – and returned to step exercises after their baby is born. The proviso here is that you must have had the all-clear from your doctor, which will be after your post-natal check-up, when your baby is at least six weeks old.

Generally speaking – and not just in pre- or post-pregnancy – if you have days where you feel less inclined to exercise (for example, at the beginning of your menstrual period, after a particularly tiring day or illness) don't feel a failure if you have to lower your step height or decrease the time or level of your step section. If you force yourself to step the whole idea will become less enjoyable and far more of a chore. As soon as you feel negatively about an exercise or diet programme you will be far less likely to persevere.

CHILDREN AND STEPPING

When it comes to children, they tend to love stepping as much as adults do. However, children cannot, in any way, be viewed as miniature adults in the context of step exercise. There are physiological and psychological differences that must be considered before you let children loose on a step programme. Young growing bodies are more susceptible to trauma than adult's bodies, therefore we cannot always expect them to manage the same exercise programme. In any case, they may not want to!

The New Stepper's and Advanced Dyna-Step Challenge, will be suitable for some fifteen- to sixteen-year-olds, and older. In fact, I find that the sixteen-year-olds that I teach, who are into their fifth week of stepping at the moment, are well able to cope with the intensity and co-ordination of the New Stepper's Challenge and are working their way up to the advanced exercises. However, children younger than this really need a specially devised step programme for maximum safety, using a low step of four to six inches, depending on their age, height and fitness levels. If your eight to fifteen year old child is keen to take part in step exercise, consider the following when you are looking for a home programme or class:

- Exercises need to be varied to retain interest. They also need to be simple. The movements need to change regularly, which may involve less repetitions of movements than in an adult's step programme. Less repetitions will mean more variety and less continuous stress on their joints. For example, rather than performing several sets of eight repetitions on one step exercise, they'd perform only one lot of eight, but go back and repeat the combination more regularly.
- Children's heart rates respond quickly to exercise, therefore they work better if their programme is intermittent; for example, they need an intense spurt of stepping for a very short period of time, followed by marching or other less strenuous movements to recover. You could adapt the New Stepper's Challenge by giving your child more breaks in between the exercises.
- Children tend to need a longer cool-down than adults to allow their heart rates to recover. Let them go for a walk around the room or the garden gradually to bring down the pace once they have finished their step routines.

- Children have shorter attention spans than adults (and I can vouch for this as a mother and ex-school teacher). They require more motivation, and the 'fun' element is important. A good step programme for children will make the steps fun; for example, like imitating football, netball or cricket movements with some of the steps.
- Stepping music may be a slower speed than for your workout. Children really need to be right down at the 118 beats per minute to step with good technique.

All of these provisos do not indicate that stepping is unsafe for children. It can be a fantastic way for them to get fit and have fun. The programmes illustrated in this book, however, are largely aimed at adult capabilities and if your child wants to join in with you, get them to do it without a step, or use a thick mat to step on and off! Anything to encourage them to adopt a healthy lifestyle! Take note, though: children should never add handweights to the exercises.

The American College of Sports Medicine recommends that our primary goal should be to encourage children to adopt lifelong exercise which will foster physical fitness and health. At present they recommend a minimum of twenty to thirty minutes of exercise. How many of our children, I wonder, actually achieve this goal? Certainly this amount of exercise is often not available in the physical education programmes in schools. We may have to look to out-of-school activities to promote the health and well-being of the future generation.

MATURE STEPPERS

At what age can we label someone as 'mature' or 'older'? Exercise programmes used to be specially devised for the 'over fifties' as this age was often viewed as the start of older age. Some fifty- to sixty-year-olds that I know would be insulted by this insinuation – and rightly so! All older adults are not the same. Just as there is no comparison between a ten-year-old and a thirty-year-old, someone who is fifty is vastly different from an eighty-year-old because of the changes in body physiology and physical ability. You cannot always categorize people by age alone because the key is the overall state of their health.

The 'young' older people (classified as being between fifty and sixty-five) are often actively involved in the community and workplace, and exercise regularly. If you are a healthy member of this age group you should have no problem with the New Stepper's Challenge, provided you observe the following points:

- Cardiovascular fitness is important, particularly in the prevention of heart disease, but as heart rates begin to lower with age, stepping should be kept at a moderate intensity. The step height should be at the low level of four to six inches.
- Flinging, jerky movements of the joints should be avoided. Get to know the exercises before putting them to music.
- Sudden turns, involving balancing skills, should be avoided. This may mean that some of the routines in the Advanced Dyna-Step Challenge will be inappropriate.
- Where a jump is offered as an option in a step sequence, it should be avoided.
- One-pound handweights may be beneficial in strengthening the upper body and may help to some degree in the prevention of osteoporosis (the degenerative bone disease that is of most concern to post-menopausal women). If these weights are used:

care and control is of major importance. You will also have been a regular exerciser in order to have the necessary strength.

Seniors (those between the ages of sixty-five and eighty) can also exercise. Exercise can be so beneficial for this age group, providing that there are no health risks. If you have not exercised for years, then stepping will be too ambitious for you. But it is not too late to take up some gentle exercise, like swimming or brisk walking, and gradually increase the level. You can increase your fitness levels at this age as well as any other age. Stepping involves a degree of balance, as you are stepping up on to a block. Bearing in mind the reducing motor skills of this group (such as balance and co-ordination), brisk walking or a low-impact aerobic class may be more appropriate and still very effective.

The benefits of exercise for the elderly are tremendous and a noticeable slowing-down of the ageing process can occur with regular exercise. We have seen so many examples in the media of 'older' regular exercisers retaining their youthful looks and vitality.

Maintaining and improving flexibility will be a primary goal which will promote an active range of motion in the joints and help people remain independent. There are sections of stretching exercises shown throughout the programme which could be used with seniors as the step can be used for support, which eliminates some of the risks involved with weight-bearing and balancing stretch positions.

If you are in this senior age group, have been stepping regularly and are intending to continue – good for you – but consider the following:

• If you develop chest pains, irregular heart rhythms or extreme breathlessness, stop at once and see your doctor as soon as possible.

- If you suffer from arthritis, do not exercise if a joint is particularly swollen or painful.
- Any signs of discomfort mean that you should stop stepping and take up more gentle exercise; e.g., brisk walking or swimming, as suggested.

Other individuals who may need 'special guidelines' before embarking on this step programme will include those people with a history of heart disease or high blood pressure, diabetics, asthmatics and anyone who suffers from joint problems caused either by disease or injury. In many cases the benefits of stepping will apply as much, if not more so, to these groups of people as to anyone else but, because there may be other implications, it is always wise to check with your doctor first. Stepping can be adapted to suit most ages and abilities which is one of the reasons why it is rapidly becoming one of the most successful exercise programmes ever to arrive in this country.

Let's make sure we safely achieve all of the wonderful benefits stepping can offer us by treating it wisely.

Step Summary

NEW STEPPER S CHALLENGE

NO. OF REPETITIONS	THE STEP	NO. OF SEQUENCE REPEATS	ARM POSITIONS (OPTIONAL)
3	Marches		
1	Heel Dig	3	Bicep Curl
3	Marches		Pec Dec
1	Toe Tap		
8	Single Heel Digs	2	Bicep Curl
8	Single Toe Taps		Pec Dec
8	March on Top of Step		
8	March on Floor	As many as	'Marching
4	March on Step	necessary	arms'
4	March on Floor		
2s	Singles, which is:		
8	Simple Steps, right lead	2	
8	Simple Steps, left lead		
4	Simple Steps, right lead	2	
4	Simple Steps, left lead		Hands on hips

NO. OF REPETIT- IONS	THE STEP	NO. OF SEQUENCE REPEATS	ARM POSITIONS (OPTIONAL)
2s	Simple Steps		
1	Step, right lead	As many as necessary	Hands on hips
1	Step, left lead, with Tap-Down Change		
8	V-Step	2	Alternating Shoulder Pull-Backs
8	Alternating Tap-Downs		
4	V-Steps	1	Front Shoulder Raises
4	Alternating Tap-Downs		
2	V-Steps	1	
2	Alternating Tap-Downs		
16	V-Step with Lunge	1	Arms overhead on the Lunge
8	Knee Lifts (alternating lead leg)		Arms overhead on Knee Lift. Pec Dec in between lifts
16	Travelling Knee Lifts	2	Shoulder Pull-Backs on leg side. Hand roll in between
8	Repeaters Knee Lifts	2	
16	Side Leg Squeezes	2	
8	Repeaters Side Leg Squeezes	2	
16	Leg Curls	2	Bicep Curl
8	Repeater Leg Curls	2	

NO. OF REPETIT-IONS	THE STEP	NO. OF SEQUENCE REPEATS	ARM POSITIONS (OPTIONAL)
8	Combination Knee Raise, Side Leg Squeeze and Leg Curl		Arms to match leg movements, as listed

FROM THE SIDE OF YOUR STEP

3	Leg Flicks Over the Top	8	Front Shoulder Raise. Breaststroke arms
3 1	Side Leg Squeeze Over the Top	8	Shoulder Pull-Backs. Breaststroke arms
3 1	Leg Curls Over the Top	8	Bicep Curls. Breaststroke arms
3 1	Combination of Leg Flick, Side Leg Squeeze and Leg Curl Over the Top	8	As above

COOLING DOWN

Do 8 repetitions of Over the Top Lengthways, gradually slowing down the pace until your breathing returns to normal.

Cool-Down Stretches
Groin Stretch, Calf Stretch, Front Thigh Stretch, Back of Thigh Stretch, Underarm Stretch, Chest Stretch.

NO. OF REPETIT-IONS	THE STEP	NO. OF SEQUENCE REPEATS	ARM POSITIONS (OPTIONAL)
	ADVANCED STEPPER S CHALLENGE		
8	Heel Digs		Bicep Curl
8	Toe Taps		Pec Dec
8	March on Top of Step		Bicep Curl
8	March on the Floor	2	Bicep Curl
4	Simple Step, right-leg lead		Hands on hips
4	Simple Step, left-leg lead		
2	Simple Step, right-leg lead		
2	Simple Step, left-leg lead	2	Hands on hips
16	Alternating Lead Steps		Hands on hips
4	V-Steps		Alternate
4	Alternating Lead Steps	2	Shoulder Pull-Backs. Front Shoulder Raises
2	V-Steps		
2	Alternating Lead Steps	2	As above
8	Travelling Knee Lifts, with optional jump		Arms over-head on lift. Pec Dec in between
3	Repeaters Knee Lifts	8	As above

NO. OF REPETITIONS	THE STEP	NO. OF SEQUENCE REPEATS	ARM POSITIONS (OPTIONAL)
8	Side Leg Squeezes		Shoulder Pull-Backs on Side Leg Raise. Hand Roll in between
3	Repeaters Side Leg Squeezes	8	As before
8	Leg Curls		Bicep Curl
3 1	Repeaters Leg Curls Combination: (Knee Lift, Side Leg Squeeze, Leg Curl)	8 8	As above Arms to go with leg movement, as already stated
3 1	Leg Flicks Over the Top	4	Front Shoulder Raises. Breaststroke arms
3 1	Side Leg Squeezes Over the Top	4	Alternate Shoulder Pull-Backs. Breaststroke arms
3 1	Leg Curls Over the Top	4	Bicep Curls. Breaststroke arms

NO. OF REPETITIONS	THE STEP	NO. OF SEQUENCE REPEATS	ARM POSITIONS (OPTIONAL)
1	Combination:		Arms to with
1	Leg Flick	4	legs, as already
1	Side Leg Raise		stated
1	Leg Curl		

FROM THE END OF YOUR STEP

NO. OF REPETITIONS	THE STEP	NO. OF SEQUENCE REPEATS	ARM POSITIONS (OPTIONAL)
8	Upside-Down V-Steps		Side Shoulder Raises
1	Diagonal Walk		
3	Knee Lifts Travelling Back	4	Arms overhead
1	Diagonal Walk		Front Shoulder
3	Side Leg Squeezes Travelling Back	4	Raises. Shoulder Pull-Backs
1	Diagonal Walk		Front Shoulder
3	Leg Curls Travelling Back	4	Raise. Bicep Curls
1	Combination: Diagonal Walk		Arms to go with legs, as
	1 Knee Lift	4	already stated
	1 Side Leg Squeeze		
	1 Leg Curl		

Repeat from the Leg Flicks through again

NO. OF REPETITIONS	THE STEP	NO. OF SEQUENCE REPEATS	ARM POSITIONS (OPTIONAL)
4	T-Steps – right lead T-Steps – left lead (optional lead)	2	Single Front Shoulder Raise

NO. OF REPETIT-IONS	THE STEP	NO. OF SEQUENCE REPEATS	ARM POSITIONS (OPTIONAL)
1	Alternating Lead T-Step (same arm as leg)	8	Single Front Shoulder Raise

FROM THE TOP OF YOUR STEP

8	Power Lunges	4	Punch arm across body. Pec Dec
4	Power Squats		
4	Turn Step		Punch single arms inside. Shoulder Raise
4	Over the Top (jump optional)		Breaststroke arms
2	Turn Steps		Same arms
2	Over the Top		Same arms
8	Alternating Turn Steps, and Over the Top (1 Turn, 1 Over the Top)		

Repeat from Power Lunges through again

Last Combination

1	Diagonal Walk		Front Shoulder Raise.
1	Turn Step		Single
1	Over the Top	4	Shoulder Raise.
2	Lunges or Jumping Jacks		Breaststroke arms

COOLING DOWN

Do 8 repetitions each of Heel Digs, Toe Taps, March on Top
of Step, March on Floor, gradually slowing down the pace so
that heart-rate returns to pre-exercise level.

Cool-Down Stretches

Groin Stretch, Calf Stretch, Front Thigh Stretch, Underarm
Stretch, Chest Stretch.

SPECIAL DYNA-STEP AND VIDEO OFFER

The Dyna-Step is distributed by Crown World Marketing and is available from all major sports' retailers at a recommended retail price of £39.99. The Dyna-Step Challenge video is distributed by Green Umbrella Productions and is available from all good video stockists at a recommended retail price of £10.99. Both can be obtained by mail order, and purchasers of this book can take advantage of the special discount offer below:

£10.00 off the Dyna-Step

£2.00 off the Dyna-Step Challenge video

ORDER FORM

Please send me:

	£	PLEASE TICK
1 Dyna-Step at 29.99 (plus £5.00 postage):	34.99	☐
1 Dyna-Step Challenge video at £8.99 (plus 50p postage):	9.49	☐
Total:	_____	

Name: _____

Mr, Mrs, Ms, Miss _____

Address: _____

_____

_____

Postcode: _____

Please make cheques payable to Crown World Marketing Ltd and send together with order form to:

Transition, Drum Grange, Nightingales Lane, Chalfont St Giles, Bucks HP8 4SL

Credit Card Hotline
Credit card holders can call **0494 764802**

Offer limited to one step per household. UK and Eire only.